I0449128

Cancer,
Thirty One Days

Eldred Krebser

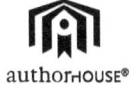

authorHOUSE®

AuthorHouse™ UK Ltd.
500 Avebury Boulevard
Central Milton Keynes, MK9 2BE
www.authorhouse.co.uk
Phone: 08001974150

First Edition published 2010 in South Africa
National Library of South Africa – Catalogued for reference
Editor Brian Andrews
Proof Reading Linda Collins, Colleen Meikle & Heather Coetzee
Cover Design Eldred Krebser © 2010
Cover Setup & Printing - C D R Repro & Print, Greyville, Durban
© 2011 Eldred Krebser. All rights reserved.

First published by AuthorHouse 1/26/2011.

ISBN: 978-1-4520-8420-6 (sc)

Nothing contained in this book is offered as medical advice and is the Authors opinion only. Please consult your General Practitioner for advice regarding any medical conditions.

The life-changing events, the fears and emotions I experienced in the "Thirty One Days" following my diagnosis with Colon Cancer.

To

Eric & Fay

My Family

My Medical Team

&

Cancer Patients Worldwide

Contents

Preface

I have spent the past twenty five years of my life in the vast outdoors of South Africa living in rural communities and basking under the African Sun.

Until my recent retirement with my partner Linda, to Durban a coastal City in KwaZulu Natal, I had been a cattle farmer in the foothills of the Drakensburg Mountains, the largest and most beautiful mountain range in South Africa. These mountains are often snow capped in the winter months, with temperatures in the region dropping to well below freezing levels, making farming conditions in those months extremely severe to contend with.

Linda and I had spent the last five years, before our retirement, isolated deep in the African Bush and far from civilization in surroundings that we thoroughly enjoyed. We had been fortunate enough to have managed the largest privately owned Wildlife Game Ranch in South Africa well positioned with a lengthy river frontage, in the Province of Limpopo. We later managed a very well known Hunting Lodge in KwaZulu Natal. Beautifully situated in the mountains of Zululand, this lodge catered for wealthy American and European Hunters and boasted many world record trophies.

The writing of this book was initially the brain child of my good friend Pete Kruger whom I met whilst both of us were recovering from surgery in hospital. Once I had started my writing, Pete would encourage me on a regular basis to keep at it. His frequent phone calls were the reason that kept me motivated in the 6 months that I needed to complete the story. Thanks to you Pete, for your constant support and encouragement, I am so grateful.

Writing this book has helped me in mentally recovering from my surgery. In a way, it has given me the opportunity to replay all the recent events of the past few months in my head and for me to try to understand and come to grips with why I had experienced such fear and emotion during that frightening journey which I had travelled.

Until my diagnosis with Colon Cancer late in 2009, I had never ever needed a consultation with a Doctor or be admitted to a Hospital during my entire lifetime. I was "Mister Healthy", never ever taking a day off work, or having to spend a day sick in bed.

This story will take readers on a medical journey that deals with my fears and emotions. To me fear was a paralyzing emotion. My greatest fear in life has always been the overwhelming fear of Hospitals, or Nosocomephobia as it is referred to in the phobia world. The thought of ever having to visit a Doctor also made me feel uneasy. In the back of my mind, I am now able to admit that I was extremely fearful of death, even though I did not express this emotion to my family at the time.

However, having experienced anaesthesia, I no longer have to think of death as an event to fear in the future. I believe the feeling one will experience when departing this life will be similar, just the final flick of a light switch and there we go, into that dark abyss.

In my opinion, after speaking to many cancer patients over the past few months and with whom I have has lengthy discussions, since having survived surgery myself, including the terrible side effects of chemo-radiation and chemotherapy treatments, I believe that cancer should be viewed as a health crisis and not as a death sentence as it is perceived by most people.

Cancer can be beaten!

Cancer is not contagious it cannot be "picked up" in the local shopping centre just as the common cold virus can. These days I feel more relaxed sitting in my Oncologists rooms where you cannot "pick up" cancer, as opposed to walking around the local shopping centre which abounds with people carrying all types of contagious germs.

I have friends that have not faced me since my diagnosis and return home from surgery. Do they belong to that group of people that believe cancer may be contagious? On the other hand, are they uncomfortable speaking to someone they think could soon die, or are they just too embarrassed to talk about the subject? They probably believe that they are immune to disease or death and live in their own fantasy world. Their time will come when they may need to face a similar situation. To satisfy my own curiosity, I will need to pursue this strange phenomenon at a later stage.

With the correct mindset and attitude, which I still needed to figure out in my own head, I had no choice but to face these fears head-on and overcome them, even though my condition may be life-threatening.

Whilst preparing to put this book together, I had read many stories relating to people suffering from the same or a similar cancer as I had. These stories came from all parts of the world. I had read stories of the incorrect diagnosis of patients in the USA, to stories of the long waiting period to get an appointment with a Specialist in the UK. This is particularly evident when a patient requires special medical investigations, as was the case with family members of mine resident in the UK.

I must therefore say, that after reading all of those different stories, contrary to the general perception regarding the state of health services in this country, it is my modest opinion that the treatment I received from my medical team in South Africa was outstanding, and must be equivalent to the best medical treatment available worldwide. The speed at which events happened was overwhelming, their diagnosis was 100% correct and I am still here to tell my story.

This is my personal story, where I share my real inner fears and emotions and it tells how I worked at overcoming them. I hope that you, the reader, finds some inspiration from my experience should you ever find yourself in a similar position.

Thanks for taking the time to read "Cancer, Thirty One Days".

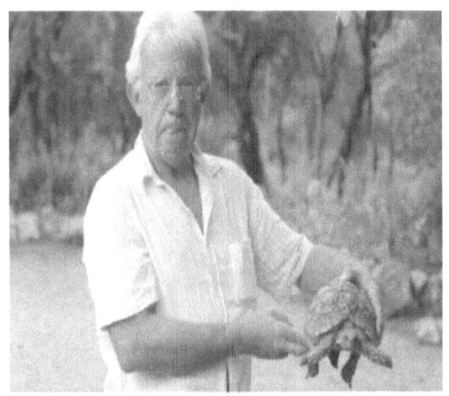

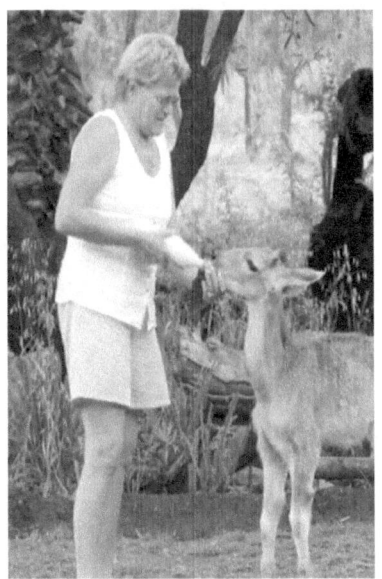

Life on a Game Ranch

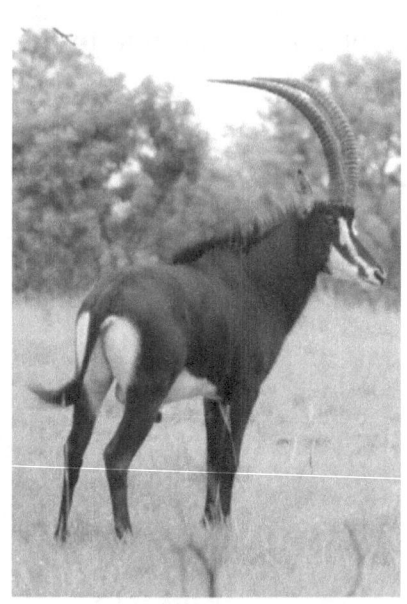

Sable Antelope

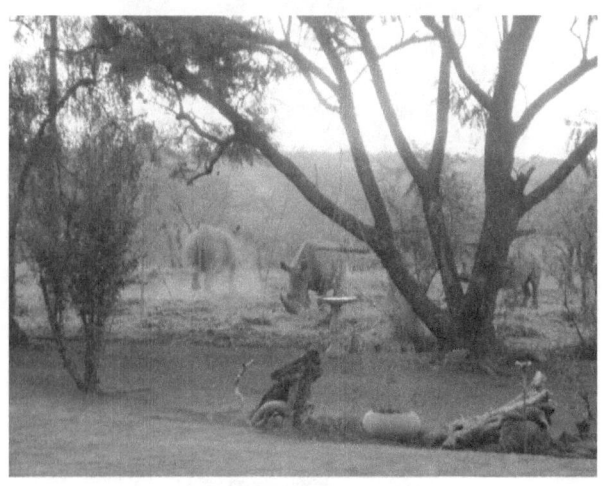

Rhino in our garden

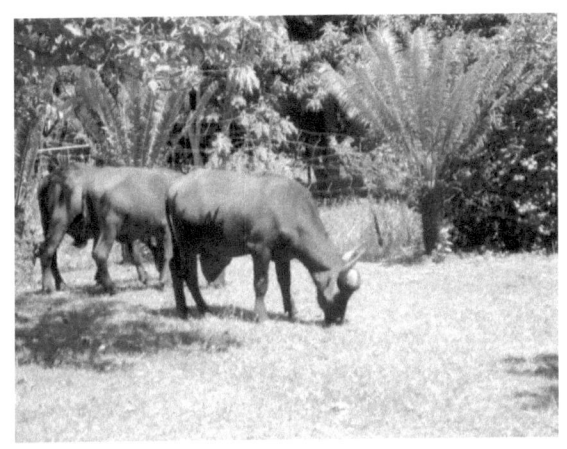

Buffalo grazing in our garden – Daughter Dawn
feeding Emma our orphaned Eland Antelope

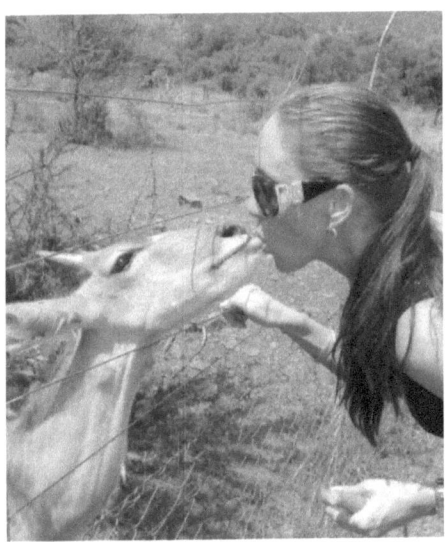

"Attitude is a little thing that makes a big difference"

Sir Winston Churchill

"Having courage doesn't imply the absence of fear, rather having courage means facing your fears head-on and overcoming them"

Larry Burkett

Author & Cancer Patient

Part One

The Build Up

Chapter One

Hospitals, not for me!

I can see the soft drizzle of rain through my bedroom windows as the wind gently moves the many beautiful white standard roses which I had pruned only six weeks earlier in our lovely garden.

It was lunchtime on Sunday, 27th September 2009, I felt very emotional and relieved to have just arrived home after a week in Hospital.

Somehow, I had managed to overcome my biggest fear in life, Hospitals. I had survived major abdominal surgery, was alive and home to start my recovery program.

Throughout my life, I have been blessed with extremely good health. This has allowed me to participate in all the sporting activities that I loved. At one stage, I was an active member of seven different sports clubs at the same time, allowing me the opportunity to participate in the highest competitive leagues and at inter-district levels. I had prided myself at being a fitness fanatic for years and just loved and lived for playing sport.

I never ever had to visit a doctor, let alone a hospital my entire lifetime. The mere thought of hospitals made me extremely jumpy and nervous and was therefore a total 'no-go' zone for me. I was so petrified of that ever happening, that I always said to my family, should the time ever come that I needed admittance to a hospital, then the medical team would need to "Dart me from a Helicopter" to get me there.

WE HAVE ABSOLUTLY NO CONTROL OVER OUR FUTURE

My time to experience the inner sanctum of a hospital had eventually caught up with me and it was with this in mind that I decided to document the series of events that happened to me during this chapter, the most traumatic and terrifying "Thirty One Days" of my life.

These events have been:

Life Threatening

Terrifying

Emotional

Fearful & Painful

Chapter Two

Warning Bells

Having been a farmer for many years, I am good at making a plan. One had to be, as the nearest town for me was 80 kilometres away. When my stomach started to play up and become irregular some weeks earlier, I made a plan. I tried every home remedy known to man, even getting the local pharmacist to dispense certain medicines. This time the plan failed helplessly and with a fair amount of pressure from my partner Linda, I sought the help of her General Practitioner, Dr Yunus Motala.

START WORKING ON YOUR MINDSET

It was Wednesday, 26th August 2009, and little did I know then, that I was about to embark on an epic journey that would take me "Thirty One Days" before I eventually returned home again. Unbeknown to me at that time, I would be minus a few body parts and would need to face a titanic mental adjustment. Many new challenges lay ahead.

CONSULT YOUR GP REGULARLY

Dr Motala is a softly spoken man with compassion in his voice. I carefully studied his credentials on the walls of his office as he questioned me about my background and previous health history.

"Yes, he was more than qualified to get my stomach up and running again", I thought to myself.

His initial check up and diagnosis made me extremely nervous. I soon realised that there was not going to be any quick fix solution to my problem here, and that all my home remedies had been in vain. Dr Motala required me to have two urgent procedures, namely a gastroscopy and a colonoscopy. The results from these two procedures would determine the cause of my internal bleeding.

I was devastated. I could see hospital looming on the horizon and immediately panic started to set in as my mind went off into a flat spin. Hospital was definitely not for me!

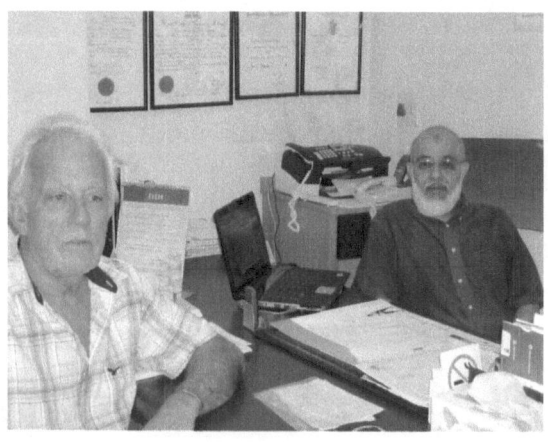

Chatting with Dr Yunus Motala my General Practitioner

FEAR STRIKES

Dr Motala did not waste any time. As I sat there talking to him, he made immediate arrangements by phone for me to meet with Dr Anver Goga, a Specialist Surgeon at the Life Westville Hospital first thing the very next morning and for the necessary procedure to be booked for the following Tuesday in the hospital day clinic.

In retrospect, I commend Dr Motala for his correct diagnosis and quick action. He has phoned me since the procedures to check on my progress and has been a great pillar of strength. I have since also visited him for a chat and we have discussed my condition and resulting emotions. He is a great caring man.

Chapter Three

Panic Stations

Preparing for these upcoming procedures was not pleasant. After drinking four litres of what tasted like rocket fuel, I felt at times that I could have launched into space! No eating is allowed for twenty-four hours prior to the procedures.

I had spent a lot of time preparing myself for this momentous hospital visit.

KEEP WORKING ON YOUR MENTAL APPROACH

I was still petrified but I had no choice, I just had to be there. I surprised myself the following Tuesday morning by actually walking into the Life Westville Hospital, without the aid of a helicopter! My knees were weak and my nerves were shot. I wanted to run, but where to?

FEAR IS A PARALYZING EMOTION

At two p.m. Dr Goga greeted me as I was wheeled into the theatre. He was very chatty as he pumped a syringe full of dope into the needle attached to my hand. Bang! I vanished into instant darkness for the following two hours.

Later that afternoon I slowly resurfaced, trying with difficulty to regain some sort of focus. Someone appeared to be feeding me a plate of sandwiches, most of which was dropping all over the floor. I later learnt it was Linda trying to feed me the sandwiches, as I obviously had no recollection of what had happened to me during that time. Unable to stand and feeling groggy, we left the hospital with Linda pushing me in a wheelchair to our car and then home for a long awaited meal.

It was the following morning that Linda and I sat nervously in Dr Goga's waiting room to hear the fate of yesterday's procedure and biopsy. My mind was in a flat spin as my heart pounded in my chest. By now I had given a lot of thought as to what may be coming and I was seriously nervous. My mind could not stop racing ahead thinking, what if? - what if?

KEEP CONTROL OF YOUR MIND

Dr Goga broke the news very calmly and sensitively. "Mr Krebser, I am sorry to tell you this. I have discovered a tumour roughly 5cm in length in your colon and from the biopsy I had taken and the test results, it is cancerous. I'm so sorry to have to tell you this bad news".

FEAR AND EMOTION TAKE OVER

My whole life froze in an instant as my brain came to a standstill. My emotions started to race, my heart was pounding in my chest and my throat was dry!

He continued, "Because the tumour is placed so far down the colon, we will need to do a full colostomy and you will need the use of a colostomy bag for the rest of your life"

A COLOSTOMY CAN SAVE YOUR LIFE!

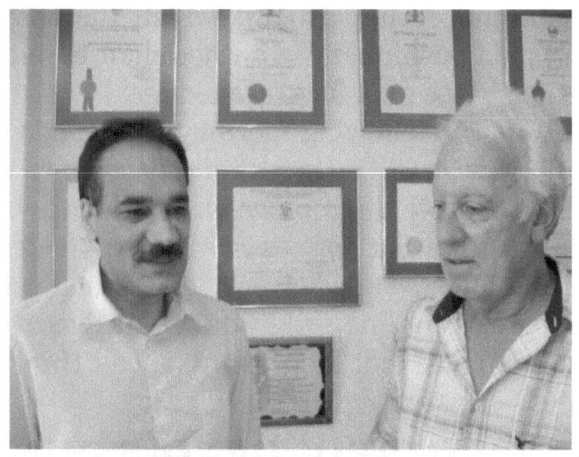

Dr Anver Goga my Surgeon & I discussing upcoming surgery

I was totally devastated. I had just been diagnosed with serious cancer of the rectum! My life flashed past me like a rollercoaster. "Was I going to die? Was I on borrowed time? What was I going to do? How was I going to cope?"

My mind was like a freight train running at full speed and totally out of control.

WORK ON YOUR ATTITUDE

Suddenly my mind flashed back some 35 odd years previously. One of my employees, who happened to be one of my neighbours at the time, had died unexpectedly one morning in hospital. It appeared that he had died from complications of a blocked bowel. In my mind, I could clearly remember and see the devastated look on his wife's face.

That picture which suddenly flashed through my mind further helped me into panic mode.

Linda and I looked at each other with tears streaming down our cheeks. Our emotions took over, as we were totally oblivious to our surroundings. I can recall at that moment my thought patterns going into what appeared to be slow motion mode, it felt like I was floating weightlessly in space and I was unable to think logically.

"Bugger this," I thought, as I tried to regain some sort of composure and to think clearly.

"What are my chances here Dr Goga" I asked.

ATTITUDE IS A LITTLE THING THAT MAKES A BIG DIFFERENCE

"From what I've seen so far, I believe it can be pretty good, however to make a proper detailed assessment I will need you to have an urgent Ultrasound and a MRI scan to determine if the cancer has spread, and if any of your vital organs have been damaged" he replied.

BEING DIAGNOSED WITH CANCER WILL SHOCK YOU INTO LIVING EACH DAY WITH A TOTAL NEW APPRECIATION TO LIFE

Once we had taken in the initial impact of this devastating news and managed to get some control over our emotions, Dr Goga showed us the pictures of the problem tumour that he had taken the day before. I remember saying to him that he might as well have shown me a picture of the surface of the moon, because that is what it looked like to me, barren and unattractive.

However to me as a layman, this tumour was not a pretty sight and was going to need some urgent intervention by someone that knew exactly what he was doing before it completely took me out.

Once again, I witnessed a doctor move with speed and purpose. Before we left his rooms Dr Goga's Secretary had made the necessary arrangements to have the Ultrasound and the MRI scans done at Netcare St Augustine's Hospital, at the earliest date available.

The results of these scans would be very important and will be used in the planning process to determine the most effective treatment method available.

Dr Goga recommended that I meet with Dr Riaz Mall, a Specialist Oncologist at the Hopelands Cancer Centre in Durban. He is a cancer specialist and well equipped to assist us further in the treatment of this dreaded disease. The necessary appointment to meet him was made by Dr Goga's secretary, Geetha.

Chapter Four

Amy to the Rescue

Linda and I walked out of the Doctors consulting rooms in a complete daze. I was completely blank and in a state of shock. "Me cancer, it can't be, it's impossible!" We were so shocked it took us an hour trying to find our car, as we aimlessly wandered around the car park together. Eventually, getting into the car Linda turned on her cell phone and made a call.

"Amy, we have just been given the results and it is not good. Please, we need your help" she said.

"I will be with you guys in 15 minutes" Amy replied.

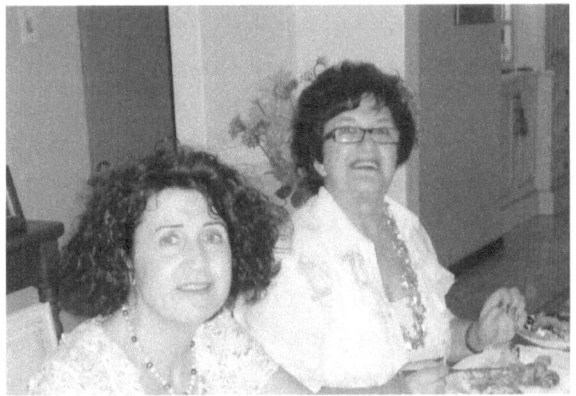

Our very good friends Amy & Colleen,
both were life-savers!

Amy is a very good friend of ours who earlier this year was diagnosed with breast cancer. She had been going through chemotherapy and radiotherapy together with their dreaded side effects for weeks. Even in her run-down condition, Amy was a lifesaver that evening. She just talked Linda and I through the shock of the day's news and kept reassuring us along the way as she took us into the dark world of cancer and our fear of that unknown road ahead. I will never forget that evening as long as I live.Thanks Amy, for all your kind and loving support and advice that frightful evening.

TALKING TO OTHER CANCER PATIENTS CAN HELP MANAGE YOUR STRESS LEVELS

The next day Linda and I decided that we needed to inform our family who now live on three different continents. Why did we need to tell them so quickly? Let me tell you why, because there was another fear hovering in the back of my mind at that time, and that was the fear of death. Is cancer not always associated with death? I had lost a few close friends over the past few years to cancer, one in particular diagnosed and gone in 90 days!

Who knows how long I was going to be around? I just needed to let all my family know the seriousness of my condition.

FAMILY SUPPORT IS VITAL

It was during the course of the following morning that the entire impact of the challenges that lay ahead and what I was about to face hit us both. Somehow Linda needed to be calm and strong as she let the family know what my diagnosis was, including that unknown road we were both about to journey down.

I was not emotionally in the right frame of mind to speak to anyone yet. I needed to first get my mind right and get some form of control over my emotions. I needed to figure out in my head how I was going to cope with a cancerous tumour in my body and the pending abdominal surgery. The thought of the chemotherapy and radiotherapy that was to follow scared me. On top of all of this was a Colostomy Bag for the rest of my life!

I needed to figure out in my mind how I was going to survive all this.

ONLY THINK POSITIVELY

I had more than enough on my mind at this point and I had no idea where to start!

ALL BATTLES ARE FIRST WON OR LOST IN THE MIND

From what I remember of that morning, Linda somehow got through all of those difficult phone calls and then fell into an uncontrollable heap.

As is the case with all families when receiving this type of horrific news, our family members were completely and utterly devastated at my diagnosis.

Chapter Five

One Step Closer

Whilst completing the necessary paper work with the receptionist in Dr Mall's rooms, I looked up to see a familiar face. It was Gavin, he had been recently diagnosed with cancer. Gavin was a sales representative with a popular vehicle agent in the town close to where I had farmed. He and I had done business together during the years that I had lived in the district and I had not seen him since leaving the area many years before.

"What a place to meet for a ten year reunion" I thought to myself.

I later bumped into Carol Kilpin, the Practice Manager, in her office a little way down the passage. I had done some work for her and her husband at their home just a few weeks earlier. What a small world we live in.

Dr Mall explained in detail to Linda and me how he proposed treating my particular form of cancer. Firstly we needed the Ultrasound results to see if the cancer had spread to any of my vital organs. If there was no spread then we were in with a good chance of beating it. After a physical examination, he was happy that there was no swelling in my liver area and that was a very good sign. He then arranged to have my Ultrasound done the following day as we needed to move quickly. Once done he could study the results and then make the necessary decisions as to how soon we should proceed with treatment.

HAVE CONFIDENCE IN YOUR ONCOLOGIST

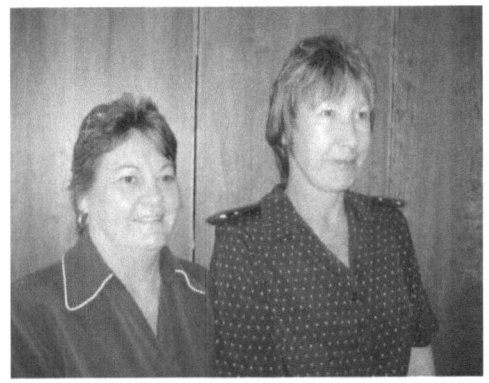

Hopelands Cancer Centre
Carol Kilpin & Sr Theresa Burrows

Blood samples were taken to measure certain levels and these would be used as a base to monitor my progress during the course of my treatment period. The best plan was to first study the results of the two scans, followed by surgery to remove the invasive tumour. Once I had sufficiently recovered from surgery there would be a series of Chemotherapy and Radiotherapy treatments. Combine these two treatments and they are referred to as Chemo-radiation.

"I will call you tomorrow afternoon as soon as I have seen your blood and ultrasound results," he said as we left his rooms.

Tomorrow was going to be the biggest day in my life. The result of the ultrasound was going to have a massive effect on my immediate future. It was going to determine whether I had a fighting chance at winning this battle or whether I was going to die!

These thoughts kept going through my mind as I drifted through the long night, unable to sleep and continually struggling with my subconscious emotions.

Trying to keep control over one's thought is not an easy task. I continuously needed to reassure myself about thinking positively all the time. At four o'clock in the morning, I got out of bed to prepare myself mentally for the "Great Unknown" day ahead.

THINK POSITIVELY ALL THE TIME

The Ultrasound took 45 minutes to complete. We waited for the Radiologist to review the scan and to have the report typed. During this time I could very easy have smoked a packet of Camel cigarettes without a problem! With surgery in the pipeline, I was pleased that I had given up this dreadful habit some months earlier.

SMOKING IS A KILLER

Whilst waiting in the reception area, I calculated that over the last 61 years of my life I had only smoked on and off for a period of six or seven years. Was that the cause of my cancer? I did not think so, but silently I had my reservations. My father had smoked up to sixty cigarettes a day during his lifetime, and had passed away in his eighties without any sign of cancer.

The sealed envelope containing the ultrasound results were handed to us by the receptionist in the x-ray department. On our way, Linda and I delivered these results to Dr Mall's rooms and proceeded home to await his dreaded phone call later that day.

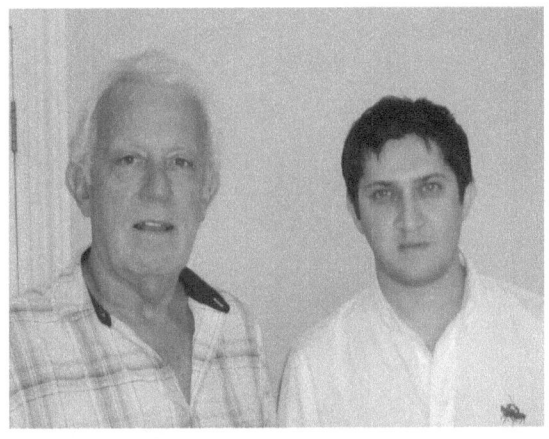

Me again, with Dr Riaz Mall my Oncologist

The rest of the day seemed to take forever, as I wondered around the house waiting for my cell phone to ring. I was trying to have a short nap when my cell rang later that afternoon. The screen showed "Private Number" and I immediately knew who was calling me. My heart began to race as it started pounding in my chest; suddenly my throat was dry as I nervously answered my phone.

"Mr Krebser, Dr Mall speaking. I have the results of your blood tests and ultrasound before me and they both look good at this stage. **Nothing has spread to your vital organs.** I want you to see Dr Goga as soon as you have had the MRI scan and then prepare yourself for surgery. Good luck and I will see you again after your surgery."

I was ecstatic with this great news!

We were now in with a fighting chance and that was just the break that I needed.

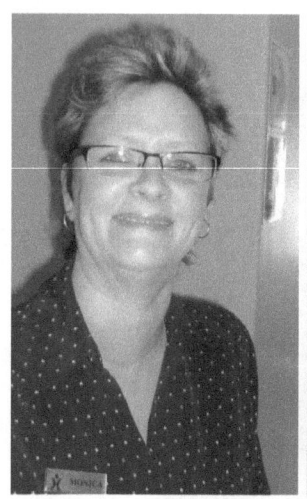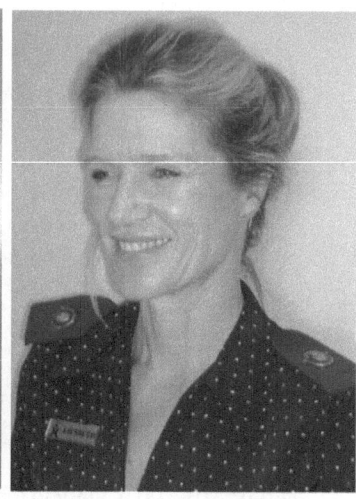

Sr Liesbeth Dawber and Pharmacist Monica Alexander, Hopelands staff

That Wednesday evening called for a celebration. Our good friend, Heather Coetzee called in on Linda to collect a parcel and left three hours later! What a great time we had that evening talking and laughing, allowing the hectic events of the past few days to disappear for a few hours.

We may have overdone things a bit that evening as I woke with a rather fuzzy head the next morning.

LAUGHTER IS A GREAT TONIC

Chapter Six
Decision Time

I needed to overcome one last hurdle, and that was the MRI scan. Once again I made a trip to Netcare St Augustine's Hospital. Some people find the noise in this machine a little too much to handle, therefore the staff recommended I insert earplugs during the scanning process.

With a slight feeling of claustrophobia, I slid into the submarine type cylinder which I did not find that uncomfortable. I closed my eyes for one hour and ten minutes as the machine ran through the necessary computer program, only stopping once for me to have some sort of dye injection administered in my arm as this would help in highlighting certain internal organs.

It was Thursday afternoon, 17th September 2009, somewhat overcast and rather cool for Durban weather this time of the year, as I waited for Dr Goga in his consulting rooms at the Lifecare Westville Hospital. Arrangements had been made for the previous day's MRI scan to be delivered directly to his consulting rooms that morning.

READ UP AND EQUIP YOURSELF WITH AS MUCH INFORMATION ON YOUR CONDITION AS

POSSIBLE, THIS HELPS WITH DECISION MAKING

Linda had a previous engagement and was not able to be with me for the first time during all our visits to hospitals and doctors consulting rooms. By now, three weeks had passed since my initial diagnosis and I had given a lot of thought to all the enormous problems ahead which I needed to face. I felt a lot more positive as I had done extensive reading on the Internet and was a great deal more familiar with my condition and confident in myself. I has studied detailed reports on the surgery that I was about to undergo. This research had given me comprehensive insight into how the surgical operation was going to proceed and what I may expect.

HAVING COURAGE DOES NOT IMPLY THE ABSENCE OF FEAR, RATHER HAVING COURAGE MEANS FACING YOUR FEARS HEAD-ON AND OVERCOMING THEM

By now, I had worked out in my mind how I was going to cope with what appeared to be this heavily stacked pack of odds against me. I needed to win, and that was my plan. If I did not win here, then I would hit the dirt just like the bad guy does in a western movie, and that was not negotiable. I had never been a loser in my entire life and was therefore not going to give up that easily. However, before I could proceed with surgery I needed the reassurance of my surgeon on one serious point.

UNDERGOING SURGERY IS A MASSIVE DECISION

Dr Goga has a very composed manner about him when he speaks to you, he leaves one feeling very relaxed and at ease. I had a list of concerns for discussion, and he encouraged me to share them with him. I explained to Dr Goga that I had in fact now realized that I needed to deal with my cancer. However the surgery and the colostomy had presented me with a much greater problem to overcome in my head. I was now a lot more at ease with these two issues since I had convinced myself of the urgency in getting this invasive tumour out of my body as quickly as possible.

"It was an easy decision at the end of the day," I said to him "I have the surgery, or else I die, it's as simple as that."

HAVE COURAGE

We spent time discussing the surgery in detail including who would make up the surgical team of professionals that would be assisting him. I was to have a procedure called an Abdomino Perineal Resection with Colostomy. In simple terms, that is the complete removal of the anus, removal of the rectum, removal of the sigmoid colon, removal of all suspect tissue surrounding the tumour area, the closure of the back passage and the construction of a stoma, or better known as a colostomy. Surgery from both the front and back will be performed at the same time.

THE THOUGHT OF SURGERY MADE ME A NERVOUS WRECK

What I found totally terrifying and needed reassurance on, was the fact that this man, whom I hardly knew, was about to cut me in half, remove half my insides, rearrange what was left in there, put me back together again and hopefully I would survive all of this to see the light of day once more. On the other hand who knows, maybe I would not?

I was scared, in fact I was petrified. For me this was going to be a terrifying journey ahead and a difficult and emotional decision to make.

Without hesitation and with a slight smile on his face, he spoke to me and took me through my fears and emotions. He gave me the reassurance that I was looking for. He was a Specialist Surgeon and was going to cure me. "God willing, all will go well," he said.

HAVE CONFIDENCE IN YOUR SURGEON

Sitting there opposite him and listening, I felt overwhelmed. I had major decisions to make within a short space of time and based on my limited information. I knew very little about cancer, even though I had done a vast amount of reading on the internet. Yet before me was this highly trained Surgeon, suggesting that he cut me in half and remove half my organs!

MAKING A SURGICAL DECISION IS A MONUMENTAL CHALLENGE

I suddenly relaxed and immediately felt comfortable enough to place my faith in this talented man as I agreed to proceed with the surgery. We agreed that Monday 21st September 2009 at one o'clock in the afternoon would be the day the surgery would take place. Two additions surgeons from the hospital, including Dr Ruwaida Khan a Specialist Anaesthesiologist, and a team of theatre sisters and staff would assist Dr Goga with the surgery

MENTALLY START TO PREPARE YOURSELF

Agreeing to undergo surgery was for me the most terrifying decision I had ever taken in my entire life!

The digestion and absorption of nutrients, as well as the storage and elimination of faecal waste, takes place within the gastrointestinal system, or the GI tract. Digestion starts in the mouth as you chew your food. Food then passes through the oesophagus to be digested in the stomach. Partially digested food moves into the small intestine, where pancreatic enzymes and bile are secreted to further break down food, and nutrients are absorbed. The remaining undigested portion thickens, as water is reabsorbed in the large intestine, or colon, forming solid faecal matter, or stool. Stool is then passed to the rectum, where it is stored until it is excreted through the anus.

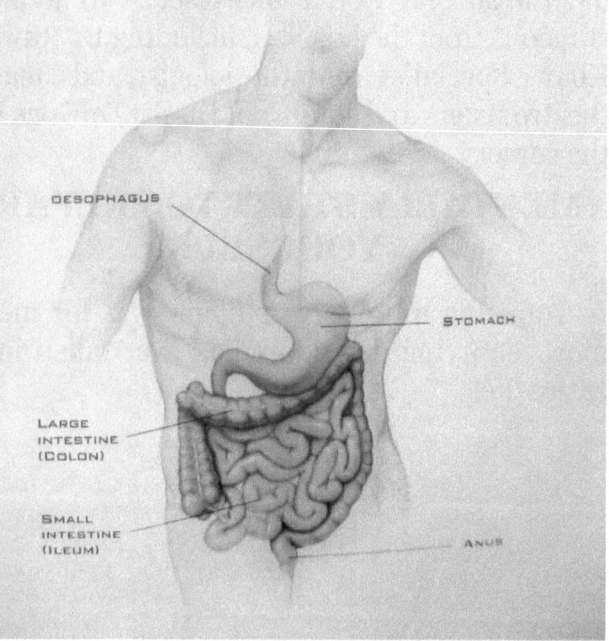

View of a healthy colon

A colostomy is a surgically created opening in the abdomen through which a small portion of the colon is brought up to the surface of the skin. This new opening, called a stoma, allows stool to pass directly out of the body, bypassing a diseased or damaged section of the colon. In some patients, this section may be removed.

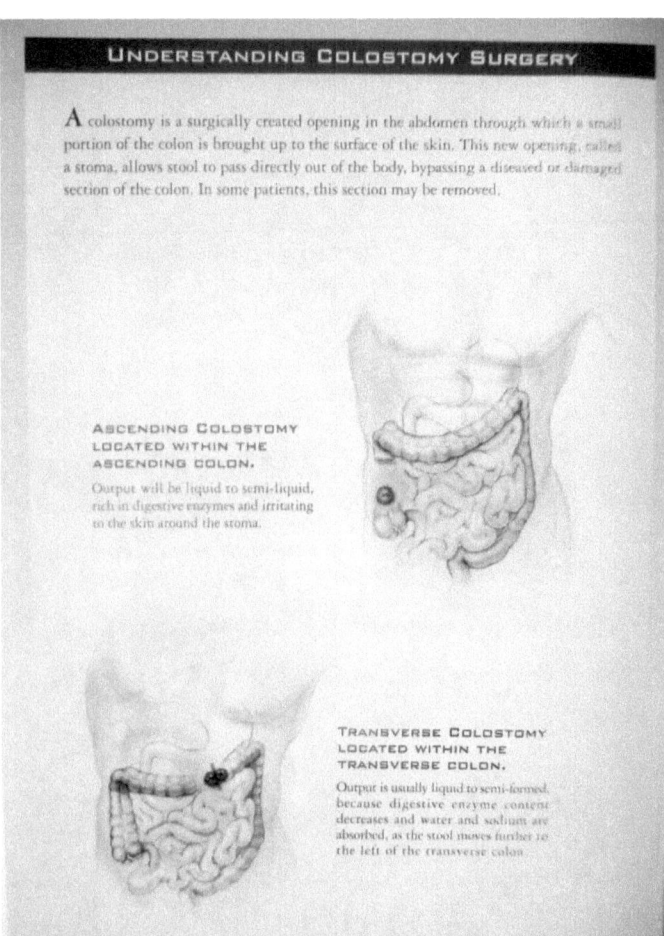

ASCENDING COLOSTOMY LOCATED WITHIN THE ASCENDING COLON.

Output will be liquid to semi-liquid, rich in digestive enzymes and irritating to the skin around the stoma.

TRANSVERSE COLOSTOMY LOCATED WITHIN THE TRANSVERSE COLON.

Output is usually liquid to semi-formed, because digestive enzyme content decreases and water and sodium are absorbed, as the stool moves further to the left of the transverse colon.

Ascending and Transverse Colostomy

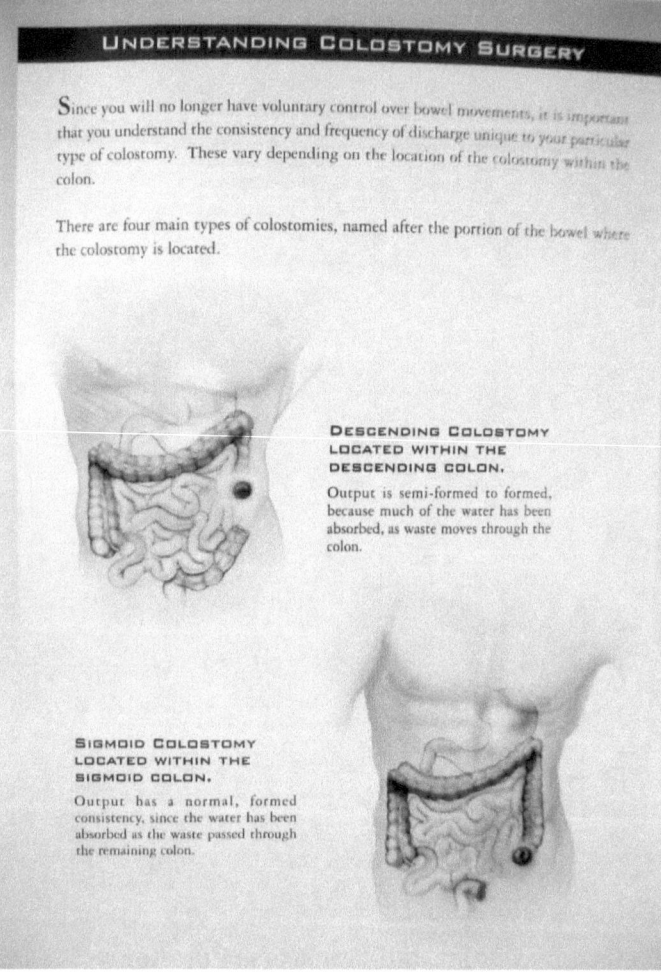

UNDERSTANDING COLOSTOMY SURGERY

Since you will no longer have voluntary control over bowel movements, it is important that you understand the consistency and frequency of discharge unique to your particular type of colostomy. These vary depending on the location of the colostomy within the colon.

There are four main types of colostomies, named after the portion of the bowel where the colostomy is located.

DESCENDING COLOSTOMY LOCATED WITHIN THE DESCENDING COLON.

Output is semi-formed to formed, because much of the water has been absorbed, as waste moves through the colon.

SIGMOID COLOSTOMY LOCATED WITHIN THE SIGMOID COLON.

Output has a normal, formed consistency, since the water has been absorbed as the waste passed through the remaining colon.

Descending & Sigmoid Colostomy, I ended up having
Sigmoid surgery

An ileostomy is a surgically created opening in the abdomen through which the end of the ileum is brought up to the surface of the skin. This new opening, called a stoma, allows waste to pass directly out of the body, bypassing a diseased or damaged section of the colon. In many cases, the colon is removed. Its function, reabsorbing water and electrolytes will be carried out to some degree by the small intestine.

After ileostomy surgery, body waste will pass through your stoma, (the opening on your abdomen), and empty into a pouch. Since you will no longer have voluntary control over bowel movements, it is important to know that the discharge of body waste will be fairly constant. Liquid or pasty in consistency, it will occur several times a day, usually after a meal.

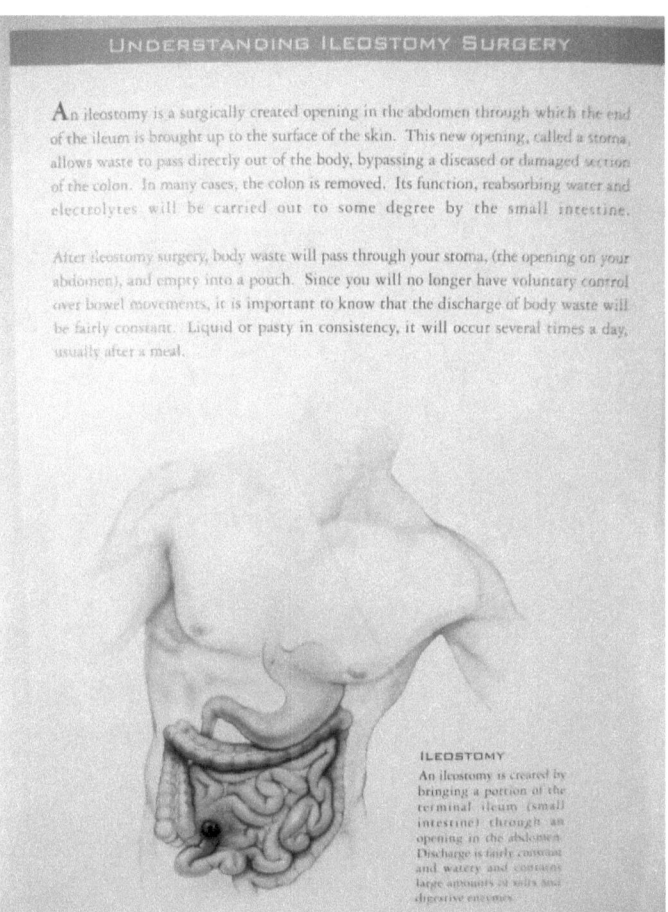

ILEOSTOMY

An ileostomy is created by bringing a portion of the terminal ileum (small intestine) through an opening in the abdomen. Discharge is fairly constant and watery and contains large amounts of salts and digestive enzymes.

Ileostomy surgery usually leads to the total removal of the colon

29

Part Two

Surgery

Chapter Seven

Fear Strikes, Surgery

I arrived home later that afternoon with the knowledge that I had four days to go before surgery. I now needed to keep control of my mind and more importantly, I had to stay busy. Sitting around and doing nothing whilst waiting for the day surgery was to take place would be a disaster. I was lucky at the time to have a few small building contracts that needed completing, so with enthusiasm and the help of one of my assistants, we got stuck in and completed the contracts by the end of the week. I was grateful that I had those jobs to keep me occupied for those few days, especially as I was not going to be able to do any heavy manual work or lift any weight in the near future. It was a huge relief to complete the work before I was out of action for the next few months.

KEEP YOURSELF BUSY

Before I knew it, Sunday had arrived and it was time to start the preparations for the following afternoon's surgery. I enjoyed a late Sunday morning brunch of pasta and salad as this was to be the last meal that I ate for the next five days. Crushed ice was the only thing to pass through my mouth during those five days in hospital. This was to allow my colon sufficient time to recover from the surgery. By the time I got home a week later, I had managed to lose seven kilograms in body weight. It's amazing how one does not get the urge for food at all and can survive for five days on a drip alone!

The next task that I needed to complete was to drink a further four litres of rocket fuel. A tip I picked up from the internet was, if the liquid is firstly chilled it would remove the foul taste and be a lot easier to swallow.

Linda and I did however have some laughter and amusement that afternoon. To save me the embarrassment of a nurse having to shave me in hospital, I got Linda to shave me from my nipples down to my knees, back and front including all the nooks and crannies. Let me tell you now, it was no fun, I did not enjoy one bit of it!

HUMOUR AND LAUGHTER CAN HELP REDUCE YOUR STRESS LEVELS

This performance is not for the ticklish type of person that I am. Linda said it felt like shaving a bear, as she needed to recharge the shaver three times before completing the job!

Monday morning arrived much faster than I had wanted. It was 4am and still totally dark outside. The date was 21st September 2009 and it was Linda's birthday. I cannot believe that I am off to hospital for surgery later today.

Looking at the clock, I thought to myself "I won't be late for this appointment, will I?"

Even though I had a restless night with my mind in turmoil, I was quite surprised to find that I had somehow managed four or five hours sleep that night.

"Here we go again" I thought, as we completed the necessary forms at the hospital admission counter. I could not believe how relaxed and calm I felt at this point. This calm however was short lived, because by the time I got upstairs to the ward I was again a nervous wreck.

KEEP CONTROL OF YOUR EMOTIONS

We entered the ward upstairs and I started anxiously chatting to the three men in the ward beds, all three were waiting for various procedures that morning. One of them was about to have a gastroscopy and was also in a state of panic.

"No problem" I tell him, "Relax it's a walk in the park," as I explain to him what to expect. One would think that suddenly I was an expert on a gastroscopy. Little did he know how nervous I was and how my heart was pounding in my chest!

He relaxed after I had explained to him what he could expect and we all laughed and joked as a carnival type atmosphere started to prevail in the ward.

PANIC STRIKES

The nurse tries to get me to get into a bed, but I point blank refuse. I suddenly want to go home! Thank goodness Linda was there to talk to me and keep me calm.

A few moments later, the ward sister arrived and wanted me to strip, put on a theatre gown and get into bed. "Don't worry" I said, "There is still plenty of time for that". The fact of the matter was that I was too scared to get into the bed. Maybe all this was just a dream and would soon go away.

"Can I go home now?" I joked, trying desperately to cover up just how weak and trembling my legs felt. I felt ill on the stomach.

"Definitely not" she replied without any humour in her voice.

Just then, Sister Irene Naidoo a theatre sister arrived in the ward. She introduced herself and asked if I would agree to her using me as a surgery case study for that afternoon, as she needed to do a detailed report on my particular type of procedure. This would help her in completing further nursing exams that she was in the process of writing. She was very grateful when I agreed to her request. I then went ahead and signed the necessary paper work. As she left the ward I got more anxious thinking that this might be much more complicated surgery than I had thought. Strange questions were going through my mind.

"What was so special about my pending procedure, why study me, could I die?"

I just could not sit still, so I kept on walking around the ward and corridors, not relaxing and unable to get into a bed.

CONTROL YOUR PANIC, KEEP REASSURING YOURSELF THAT ALL WILL GO WELL

Dr Ruwaida Khan, Specialist Anaesthesiologist arrived in the ward and introduced herself to me. We spent some time discussing my medical history and the upcoming procedure. She explained about giving me an epidural anaesthetic in my spine for a start, as this would give her far better pain control management during surgery. A further general anaesthetic would complete the knock out.

At the thought of "Pain", I got more nervous. We shook hands and I wished her the best of luck for her part in the surgery ahead.

In walked another woman who introduced herself as Sister Jocelyn Taylor, and told me that she was to be my "Stomatherapist". Dr Goga had told me about her and that she would call on me before surgery commenced. Jocelyn very quietly and calmly explained to us in detail the way in which a colostomy works.

She then proceeded to accurately measure where my Stoma would exit on my abdomen and marked the correct position with a pen so that Dr Goga knew exactly where to make the new opening. Jocelyn would visit me after surgery in the ward and guide me on "Living with confidence after Colostomy Surgery".

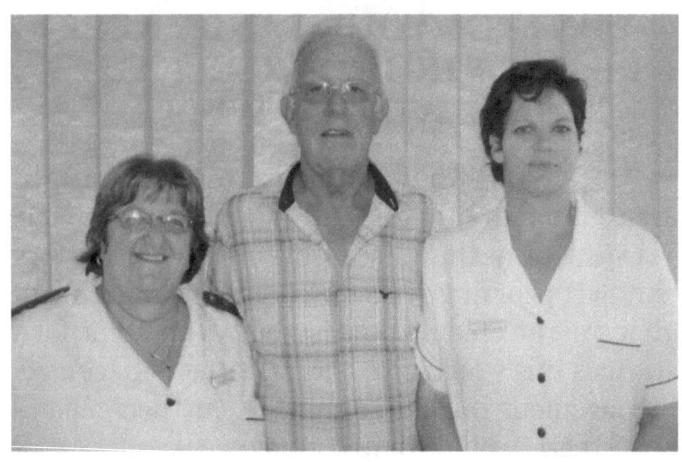

My Stomatherapy Team Sr Pam Welch and Sr
Jocelyn Taylor

My surgeon Dr Goga with his usual smile
arrived in the ward. "Mr Krebser, you are going
to be just fine, don't you worry about a thing. I
will see you in theatre in a few minutes time". We
shook hands and I wished him well for the surgery
ahead.

The ward sister together with the help of a nurse
eventually cornered me and got me to strip. I put
on a theatre gown and got into a bed. They then
administered a premed drug which is supposed to
calm one down for the trip to the theatre. I should
have had a double dose of premed two hours ago
when I got there. Maybe a double whiskey may
have even done the trick?

FEAR IS A PARALYZING EMOTION

My emotions are now hopping around like you
cannot believe. As we enter the lift on our way

to the surgical unit, I lay on the trolley thinking about how I was supposed to be darted from a "Helicopter" and wondering how I had managed to end up here without the help of one. Linda was with me, holding my hand like a little school boy, as we entered a room full of patients awaiting surgery.

"This room looks like a pre-op parking lot" I thought to myself.

If Linda had the chance she would be into the theatre with me, I know her too well. The thought of waking up with nausea suddenly scares me. As the staff wheeled me into the theatre, I said goodbye to Linda. I then said a quick prayer, which I am not very good at doing.

FACE YOUR FEARS HEAD-ON AND OVERCOME THEM

I am now actually in a sitting position on the theatre table, with my legs down the side and my feet on a stool. I cannot believe I'm doing this! Dr Khan chats to me as she prepares the epidural that she is about to insert into my spine. Now, with the premed having kicked in I was feeling completely relaxed and I still could not believe where I was or what I was doing. I watched the activity in the theatre with great interest, trying to take in as much information as possible as the theatre staff prepared the unpacking of various sterile packs of equipment to be used by the medical team during surgery.

I thought to myself, "With all these surgical tools about and the strong lights above, it looks very much like my workshop at home. Maybe we could have done the job there?"

Next moment - Bang, like a rifle shot, Dr Khan has inserted the epidural, pressed the button and away I slipped into a black abyss for the next 4 hours and 46 minutes. She had mentioned before the surgery that it would be a lot more comfortable for me to awake from the anaesthetic with all the necessary pipes removed from my nose and throat, before moving me to the Intensive Care Unit. This appeared to be happening as I slowly drifted through the mist able to hear voices but not able to focus.

I could hear Dr Goga's voice somewhere in the distance. "The surgery has been a complete success," he was saying to someone.

Laying there I thought to myself, "I must still be alive?" as I drifted off once again into darkness for the next 10 hours.

If you have never experienced this before, then I must tell you that waking up in the Intensive Care Unit for the first time was a scary experience. I was groggy and half-asleep, I had no idea where I was and there was this bright overhead light shining into my eyes. As I slowly focused, I looked down across my chest to find that I was stark naked with a Nursing Sister giving me a nice warm bed-bath."Good morning Mr Krebser, you have come through your surgery extremely well" she said.

"Good morning, any chance of covering me please, this is most embarrassing" I replied.

As my mind cleared, I could see and feel the array of pipes and tubes attached to me. I had pipes and tubes into and out of every opening in my body. Where I was short of an opening, a new one was made. In total at one stage, there were 10 tubes and pipes sticking out of my body!

Luckily, as each day passed and I slowly improved and got stronger, the nursing staff systematically removed the pipes, drips and drains. This made moving around in bed so much easier and more comfortable.

TALK YOURSELF INTO RECOVERING QUICKLY

The next two days consisted of steadily recovering whilst drifting in and out of sleep. "Morphine must be a wonderful drug" I thought, as I often pondered at the lack of pain I felt after such major surgery.

For me the pain I suffered in the areas in which the surgery took place was truly minimal. I had certainly expected a lot worse. Morphine, I am told can also make patients hallucinate to varying degrees. Once having decided to document the month's events following my diagnosis, the thought of calling my book "Eldred in Wonderland" often went through my mind. This thinking could only have come from the side effects of morphine.

The most difficult thing for me to do in bed each day was to turn onto my sides for the physiotherapist to pummel my lungs from the back. Once this physiotherapy treatment was completed, one needed to finish the exercise by having a big cough. The coughing was to help get rid of phlegm on the lungs. For me this was a difficult task to do, as coughing was not that easy and rather painful, it felt as though I was going to pop all the staples holding my stomach together. The object of this exercise was to make sure I did not end up with pneumonia. To help prevent blood clots from forming, I had to wear elastic stockings on both legs for a few days.

I cannot praise the sisters and nursing staff of the Intensive Care Unit enough, for all the care and attention I received 24 hours a day. Their dedication to caring for the sick and recovering patient is outstanding and I issued each one with an imaginary "Gold Medal" as I left the Intensive Care Unit and was moved to a General Ward upstairs. I had been in their constant care for two and a half days.

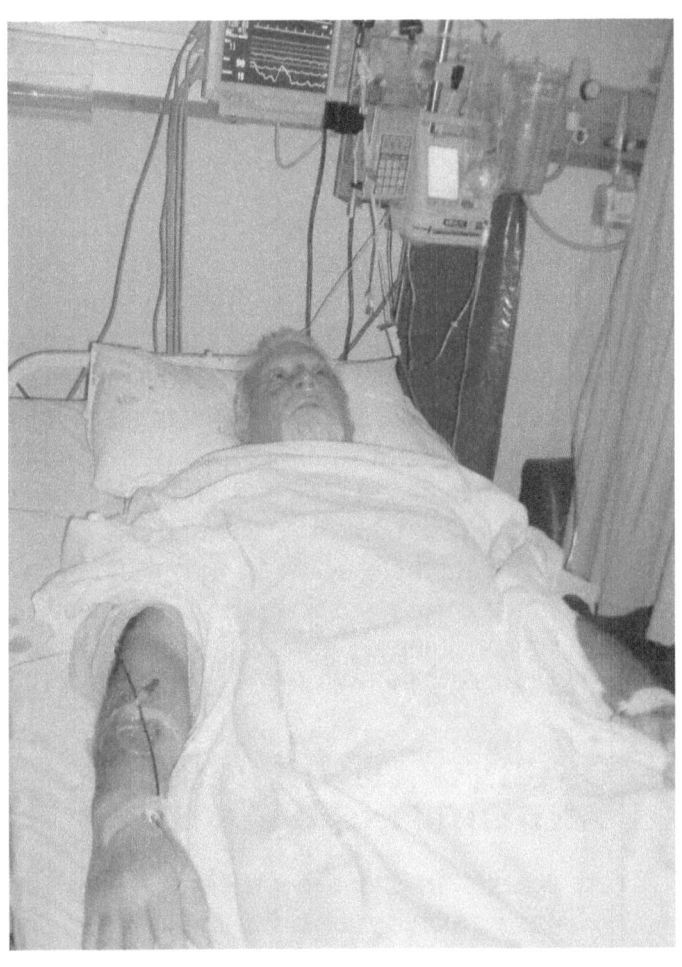

That's me recovering in Intensive Care Unit

Chapter Eight

I have Survived

It was a good feeling to be wheeled into a General Ward after those two and a half days in I.C.U. I got the feeling that I was getting well and was worthy of this promotion to a general ward upstairs. I had made it to the next level on my road to recovery.

I cannot stress enough, the importance of how this move upstairs did wonders for my emotional and psychological well-being. I often found myself in I.C.U. having all sorts of strange thoughts, probably with the help from the morphine in my system. For me this was just the right place to concentrate on keeping a very positive mindset for my recovery. Moving out of I.C.U. was a big bonus!

CONCENTRATE ON RECOVERY AND GETTING BACK HOME

Pete Kruger in the bed opposite me in the general ward greeted me with a big smile as the nurse wheeled me in. His face was so familiar, but as it later turned out we had never met before.

During the past year Pete had a bad time with his one leg, eventually succumbing to amputation below the knee, due to bad circulation. While coming to grips with this huge adjustment in his life, he suffered the same problem with his other leg, losing that one as well. This man has such courage. He heartily welcomed me to the ward.

In the bed next to Pete was Jerome Moses. Jerome was suffering with the after effects of very severe Viral Encephalitis. This disease starts in the brain and slowly shuts down one's entire nervous system to the point where you could die. Jerome had been teetering on the brink of death and luckily for him was slowly on the mend, thanks to the determination of his astute wife Amina, and a fast thinking Doctor. That's another story on its own.

I introduced the two of them to Linda and my "Board Meeting" concept, which the two of us have used for many years. Each morning during breakfast, we would discuss our plans for the day ahead. Later that day over dinner, we would review the day's progress and if necessary we could make any change or updates to our progress. The two of them thought that to be a good idea, so we put the basic plan into practice. Each morning at around 4am when we were woken, our early morning "Board Meeting" would begin. The only items eligible to appear on the daily agenda was to motivate and support each other, including our plans ahead for our full recoveries.

I will never forget those many long hours of discussion among the three of us.

THE POWER OF POSITIVE THINKING WORKS

There is no doubt in my mind that those daily Board Meetings helped us all a great deal in coping with our individual emotions, culminating in our recovery and speedy return home.

We have all since left hospital and look forward to our next Board Meeting, which we will hold at one of our homes. I hope that all three of us will be strong enough to attend and to be able to discuss and celebrate our continued recovery and good health.

One matter that does need mentioning was meal times in hospital. I have never had a problem eating and I really enjoy good food. By the time I reached the General Ward, I had not seen a decent meal in days and was now starting to look forward to one once more. When it eventually arrived, all I got was soft-type meals like jelly and custard, bananas, chicken soup and soft pastas. It reminded me of my days in the army. What a letdown, but it is common knowledge that hospitals are generally not renowned for their culinary expertise. I guess your meals in hospital are dependent on your condition at the time. It was good to later get home to Linda's great home cooked meals.

It was always great to have family and friends visit me during those recovery days. I can clearly remember one of those days when two of our staff members came with Linda to visit me. Neither of them had ever seen the inside of a hospital before and they both looked overwhelmed at what they saw. At the end of the visiting hour, they asked if they could pray for me. There I lay, with all of us holding hands as one of them prayed aloud, unperturbed by the presence of the other patients in the ward. I found this to be an emotional moment that I shall never forget.

I had many other emotional moments during those days of recovering, as the morphine slowly worked its way out of my system. One of those moments related to the following incident. Until such time as you were able to get out of bed, walk unassisted to the shower and shower yourself, there was no going home.

Jerome had managed to walk three or four steps one morning with the help of his physiotherapist and a walking aid. He had great difficulty walking as he had been flat on his back for quite some time. As he made it back to his bed I could see the strain on his face. His legs were trembling and he was as white as a sheet. Unbeknown to me, my turn was coming the next morning.

DO THE DAILY EXERCISES YOUR PHYSIOTHERAPIST GIVES YOU

The following morning my physiotherapist assisted me into a sitting position next to my bed, while she pummelled my lungs from the back. I was terrified of getting pneumonia, as my mother's sister had died of that complication in hospital after having surgery a few years back. That incident kept reminding me that I needed to get the hell out of this place as quickly as possible, away from all these sick people and the germs associated with hospitals. I needed to get home fast!

Helped into a standing position and holding onto a walking aid, I was ready to go. Crash, down I went into a heap. I was unable to lift either of my legs and could not stand alone unassisted! My legs would not work or carry my weight. That incident was devastating for me. With help from the nursing staff, I made it back into bed and spent the rest of the day feeling very down and depressed.

Thanks to Pete and Jerome who both kept encouraging me, they kept me going that day. I decided to concentrate on doing my leg exercises in bed for the rest of the day.

"I must walk, I must get out of here," I kept telling myself.

KEEP WORKING ON YOUR STATE OF MIND

It was 2am the following morning and Sister O'Sullivan had just been on a ward round to check on the three of us. I was wide awake, unable to sleep and replaying the day's events in my mind, when suddenly I had a huge emotional wobbly. There I was, 61 years old and for the first time in my life I was unable to walk or stand alone unaided. What a disaster that was for me.

That morning's event made me think of my son Bruce, now married with two children. Bruce was born with Cerebral Palsy and we had taught him to walk with the assistance of crutches from the age of three.

Bruce had never been able to walk or stand-alone unaided his entire life!

NEVER, NEVER, NEVER, GIVE UP.

KEEP ON FIGHTING FOR YOUR SURVIVAL

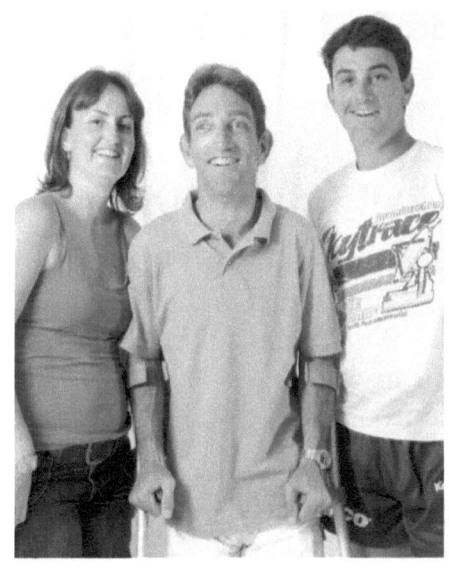

Bruce with his brother & sister,Wayne and Debbilee

As I lay there in the early hours of the morning, emotional and with tears streaming down my face, I thought of how brave and courageous my son had been throughout his entire life!

The following day I was determined to improve on my first morning's attempt at walking. After yesterday's failed shot, I was the topic of discussion in the ward for the morning and had attracted an audience to watch me, as I attempted my second walk! Once again with the aid of my walker and my physiotherapist I stood up, took a deep breath and with wobbly legs took my first step, then another, then another.

Pete and Jerome were cheering me on and so were the rest. I then lifted the walking aid and carried it, as I made off down the passage way to the delight of all. I was so determined.

"Keep walking, keep walking," I kept telling myself. I was away and nobody was going to stop me now!

PUSH YOURSELF TO THE LIMITS

The following morning I managed to walk to the showers unassisted and have my first shower in a week. What a fantastic occasion that was. I managed to walk back to my bed without any assistance from the nurse. I felt thrilled and was so proud of myself.

GET WALKING AS SOON AS POSSIBLE AFTER SURGERY

It was Saturday morning and Dr Goga had heard of my walking saga from the ward sister. After chatting to me, he was very pleased with my progress. "If you feel good and are confident with yourself, you can go home tomorrow" he said.

LISTEN TO YOUR BODY

That was good news to my ears. It was a good feeling to be going home tomorrow after a week in hospital. I was alive and well and could not wait to get home.

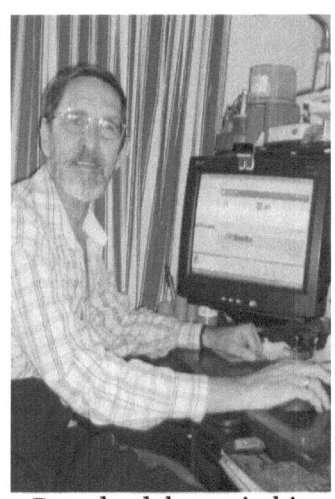

Pete, back home in his office.

It was an emotional moment for me as I said farewell to Pete and Jerome with a handshake and some sadness, as I prepared to leave the ward in a wheelchair for my journey home. The three of us had become good friends over the past few days and had shared many stories and emotional moments.

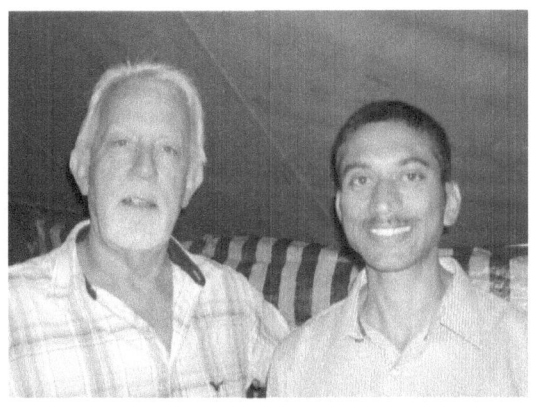

Jerome and I at his 42nd birthday celebration

"Now you buggers, you both get well soon and get the hell out of here quickly, there is a Board Meeting coming up in a few weeks time and I need you both to be there!" I said, as Linda and I headed home.

Chapter Nine

Home at Last

It was lunchtime Sunday 27th September 2009 and I was looking through my bedroom window at the gentle falling rain. I was still feeling very emotional, but I was home at last. I had overcome my biggest fear in life, Hospitals.

With determination, I had managed to keep my mind on my goal, which was with the correct attitude and mindset, to survive abdominal surgery. I was alive and feeling well and ready to start my recovery program.

IT'S ALL IN THE MIND

It had taken me "Thirty One Days" to return home.

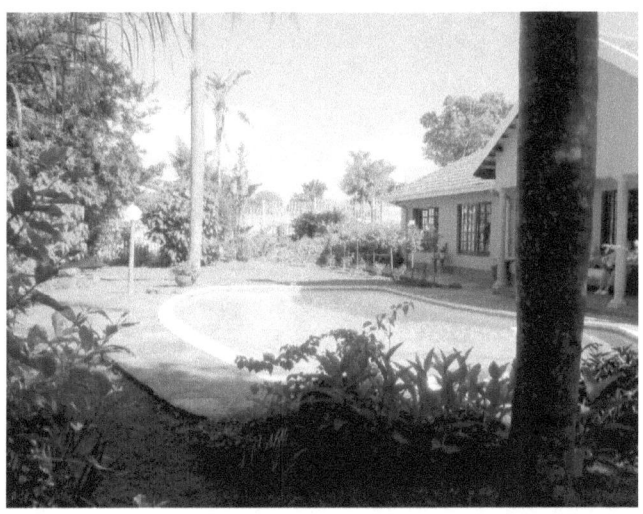

The right place to start my recovery, in our beautiful garden

Part Three

Chemotherapy & Radiotherapy

Chapter Ten

Getting Stronger

It was now Monday 5th October 2009 and I had been home one week and was really feeling great. I felt well rested and was on my way to a speedy recovery.

My first few days at home did however present me with a problem. I could not get out of bed! Beds at home are a lot lower than in hospital, so I found it difficult to sit up without help. No problem, to overcome this I would call for Linda or one of our staff members to lend a helping hand to get me up into a standing position.

EXERCISE YOUR BODY

Luckily for me I rapidly improved and was able to get myself in and out of bed without assistance by the end of the first week.

In an effort to get stronger and more mobile again, I drew up a walking plan. From day one, I would walk from the bedroom to the far end of the house and back, steadily increasing this distance daily. By the fourth day I was walking around the garden and the swimming pool area, with a bit of assistance. The more I walked, the better I felt. I needed to get my strength back and walking was certainly doing it for me.

GOING HOME WITH A NEW DISPOSAL SYSTEM ATTACHED CAN BE DAUNTING

Sister Jocelyn Taylor, my stomatherapist, had been a great help. Since surgery, she had visited me in hospital daily and has since done a few house calls. She guided and advised Linda and I on living with confidence after colostomy surgery, and we could now both cope with the day-to-day maintenance of a stoma and colostomy bag without any problem whatsoever. That Monday Jocelyn removed all the metal staples and other stitches in my abdomen, it felt great with them removed, I could now move around a lot more freely.

LEARNING TO COPE WITH A COLOSTOMY BAG IS EASY

It was a week later when a far more relaxed Linda and I were sitting in Dr Goga's rooms. We were there for my first consultation to check on my progress since leaving the hospital two weeks earlier. The circumstances had now changed from our first visit here, and it felt a bit like a reunion get together, as the three of us greeted each other, with handshakes all round.

By now I had put together some thoughts about my experience and presented Dr Goga with my first unedited version of "Cancer, Thirty One Days". He was overwhelmed at receiving my story and said he would treasure it, as he had never before received anything like it from a patient. Was that the reason why I passed my physical examination with flying colours? My examination showed that all the surgery had healed and my condition was excellent. I attribute this to the great work Dr Goga had performed on me together with my correct mindset for a positive and speedy recovery.

An appointment for me to meet with my Oncologist Dr Mall, in two days time was booked, as we now needed to prepare for the next part of my journey.

Happy with the result of our visit to Dr Goga, we decided to stop on our way home to visit both Pete and Jerome, my hospital mates and update them with my progress. Neither of them knew we were coming, so what a pleasant surprise for Jerome and Amina his wife when we walked in on them unexpectedly. What a lovely welcome we received from them. We received the same reception when we called on Pete at his home a little later that same morning. It really was good to chat to them all while catching up on our varying health issues and degrees of progress.

SURROUND YOURSELF WITH QUALITY FRIENDS WHO CARE

As we were all responding so well and on the road to recovery, we agreed unanimously that the time was now right to convene that "Special Board Meeting" we had discussed in hospital. We decided that this meeting would be held during the following week at Pete's home.

Chapter Eleven
Dynamite in my Body

I consulted with my Oncologist, Dr Riaz Mall two days later to discuss my post operative condition and how he proposed handling my cancer treatment. He had already heard from Dr Goga since the completion of my surgery and had put together a plan of how my particular treatment program would look.

We were now able to spend time discussing the finer details of this plan. An appointment had been booked for the following week, at the Netcare Parklands Hospital Radiotherapy Section, for my planning session to be done. This planning session was for the radiotherapy treatment which was about to start. The full results of this planning session would be sent to Dr Mall for his final approval and then the treatment could begin.

We discussed the possible side effects that may occur once commencing with the Chemo-radiation. Firstly with Radiotherapy, the most common problems that I could expect were redness to the skin in the treatment area, much like sunburn but progressively becoming darker, together with this was the likely loss of hair in the treatment area only. I should avoid excessive exposure to direct sunlight at all times as one's skin becomes extremely sun-sensitive.

USE LARGE AMOUNTS OF SUNBLOCK

A suitable sun block lotion must be applied at all times when exposed to excessive sunlight. Since my radiotherapy began, I have experienced the effects of exposure to excessive sunlight and it is not at all pleasant. Serious skin allergies will appear and itching will become prevalent.

If the bladder was in the direct treatment area then I would probably experience a burning sensation when urinating. During my treatment period this did become a very unpleasant painful daily occurrence, but luckily it disappeared quickly and I was back to normal within three days of completing my last treatment.

DRINK PLENTY OF LIQUIDS

It was strongly recommended that the entire region that was going to be exposed to radiotherapy be kept completely dry throughout the course of the treatment period. Getting the treated area wet and directly applying bath soaps, could lead to serious skin conditions including blistering and peeling, which could become very painful. To avoid any unnecessary inconvenience later, I decided not to shower for the duration of the treatment period. Logic told me that it would have been impossible to keep the entire treated area around my midriff dry while trying to shower each day. I would now have to shower in the bathroom basin for the next five weeks! Now there was something to look forward too!

WITH THE SIDE EFFECTS, I CONVINCED MYSELF THE CANCER CELLS WERE BEING OVERWHELMED

The side effects of chemotherapy could have been a lot worse. Nausea and vomiting, diarrhoea, constipation, bladder infection, loss of hair, sores in the mouth, hand and foot syndrome and bone marrow suppression which is low blood count, making one more susceptible to infection. Staying away from sick people during your chemotherapy treatment is highly recommended.

AVOID SICK PEOPLE TO REDUCE THE RISK OF INFECTION

My treatments were to consist of 25 sessions of radiotherapy on a daily basis from Monday to Friday. On Saturday and Sunday you are able to give your body a break and allow your system a short time to recover.

Coupled with the radiotherapy would be a course of chemotherapy, consisting of Xeloda Chemo tablets to be taken orally after breakfast each morning. These tablets are normally used in the treatment of advanced breast cancer in women, but are known to give good results in my particular type of cancer. "Chemo-radiation" is the name given to this combination of treatments.

From the day I first visited my General Practitioner up until the day I returned home following surgery, that part of my journey had taken me "Thirty One Days". I was amazed to calculate that my course of chemo-radiation was going to take exactly the same time to complete, "Thirty One Days". I needed 25 treatments plus 3 weekends, that's 31 days. After completion I found that I had displayed a total of "Thirty One Pictures" in the book. This was quite mystifying to me.

Ashni Royan is a Radiotherapist at Netcare Parklands Hospital and was going to be responsible for the set-up and planning session for my radiotherapy treatment. Before the actual set-up began, she spent some time explaining the procedure I would be following. Firstly, certain important indem-nity

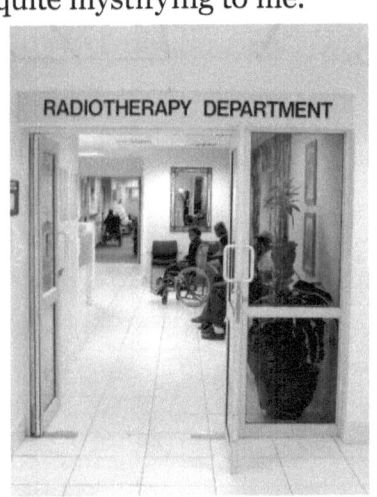

I did 5 weeks of Chemo-radiation here!

paper work needed signing, as this covered the dangers of the proposed treatment. She spent time counselling me on the side effects I may experience during treatment. I had already discussed all the negative side effects with my Oncologist and had found and read all the relevant information on the internet.

Up until that meeting with Ashni, I had never given a thought to any other cancer patient's fears or emotions, which they may have experienced during their treatment period. It had not occurred to me in the least,

I had been completely engrossed in my own little world. It suddenly hit me then, that many cancer patients are not able to cope emotionally with their condition and that they could be in desperate need of help and counselling support. Why had I not thought of this?

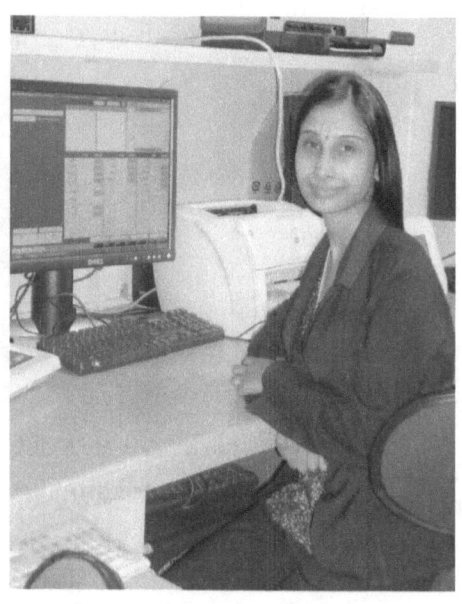

Ashni Royan did the planning of my Radiotherapy treatments

JOINING A SUPPORT GROUP WILL IMPROVE YOUR QUALITY OF LIFE

On my next visit, as I passed through the reception area I discovered a large amount of informative flyers and brochures available on display for those patients needing that support.

"My book may be helpful one day to cancer patients," I thought to myself while browsing through the display.

A SUPPORT GROUP WILL ALLOW YOU TO DISCLOSE AND DISCUSS ALL YOUR FEARS AND EMOTIONS

Next was a trip to the CT scanner, this time in the Radiology Department, but firstly I had to drink a litre of special liquid spaced over a period of one hour, closely followed by an intravenous dye injection. This injection was to identify and record the exact position of certain internal organs using the latest sophisticated computer technology. These results are then used in determining the best and safest way to deliver the radiotherapy treatment.

My body position was altered on numerous occasions whilst lying in the CT scanner and was finally set into the correct position. I had to lie motionless for some time as the radiotherapist could then mark my stomach with permanent tattoos. This is to ensure that only the marked areas will be exposed to radiotherapy treatment each day when using the Linear Accelerator Machine.

The final set-up results were sent to Dr Mall for further planning and approval. Once finally approved I was able to commence treatment within fourteen days. Great care is taken that no vital organs are damaged during the upcoming treatment and emphasis is placed on double-checking all the calculations related to the set-up, as the radiotherapy team work to tolerances of within one millimetre. A strict quality assurance program is in place to monitor the system.

It was Wednesday 4th November 2009, and I was about to start my chemo-radiation treatment at Netcare Parklands Hospital. I had taken my first dose of Chemo tablets and my blood samples had been taken in Dr Mall's rooms earlier that morning. I was now ready for the next step in the process.

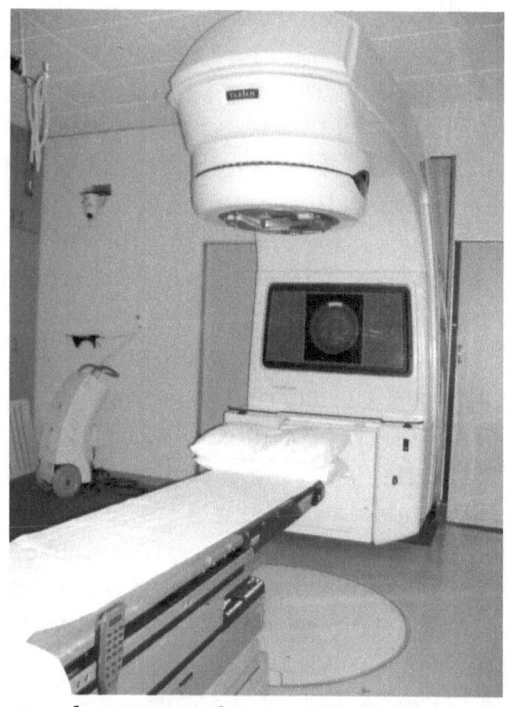

Linear Accelerator Machine - a Radiation Generating machine used for the treatment of tumours

The look of a Linear Accelerator Machine was rather daunting as I lay down on it for my first treatment to commence.

Each treatment would be supervised by a team of highly competent radiotherapists, in my case lead by Tina Owen and Merridy Hawkins. Once I had been correctly positioned and aligned by the computer model and carefully marked with paint on my stomach and sides, along the lines where I had the CT scan, I was given my first blast of an 18 megavolt dose of radiotherapy. This procedure was done on all four sides of my midriff.

There is nothing to fear here, as the treatment is totally painless.

DONT BE INTIMIDATED BY THE LOOK OF A LINEAR ACCELERATOR MACHINE

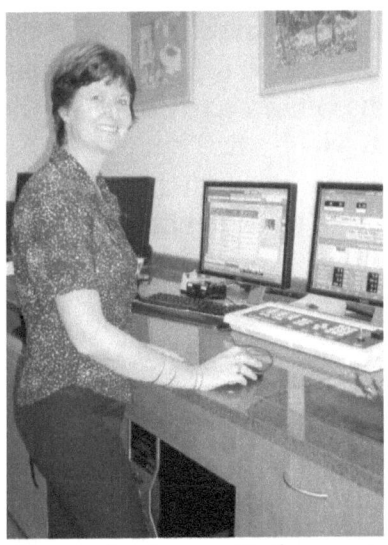

Tina Owen supervised my radiotherapy treatments

The machine rotated in a circular motion starting on my right side, and then moved to my front, then left side and finally my back. This procedure would continue daily for twenty-five days and it would take approximately five to eight minutes per session to complete.

Each new week would begin with a visit to my Oncologist's rooms in order to collect the following week's chemo tablets and at the same time have blood samples taken for testing. These blood results will be closely monitored and if needs be could lead to my medication dosages being changed accordingly. A quick consult with the Doctor determined whether I was progressing well or not.

Luckily for me I coped exceptionally well during my treatments and showed no serious side effects. The few minor problems that I faced were manageable on my part with very little discomfort. The chemo tablets did however cause me a fair amount of discomfort particularly in the diarrhoea department, which I had known might happen.

As a new recruit with a colostomy bag, I had no option but to learn to handle the situation very quickly!

ATTITUDE IS A LITTLE THING THAT MAKES A BIG DIFFERENCE

I assure you, living with a colostomy bag is no big deal. Once you have your mind around having to cope with this new accessory, it is not that difficult to adapt too. At times it may be a little inconvenient to you, especially at a dinner party or a shopping centre, but one soon learns how to cope, you have no choice!

Chapter Twelve
Finally

Shortly after starting my chemo-radiation I got a call from my Surgeon late one morning, requesting a special favour. Sitting opposite him in his consulting rooms was a patient that showed similar symptoms of the cancer that I had been diagnosed with.

This poor man was devastated with his diagnosis and was reluctant to proceed with colon surgery as he first needed to speak to someone who had previously gone through the same situation.

"Would it be possible for him to speak to you?" asked Dr Goga.

"No problem at all, send him up right now if you like, I'm home at present and I will give him as much help and encouragement as I can" I replied.

The patient, together with his wife and brother, were with me in twenty minutes. From his face, I could see where I had been a few weeks earlier, terrified!

After many questions and a lengthy discussion, they left me an hour later, all feeling a lot more comfortable and well informed. Their fear of that unknown road that lay ahead had been made clearer, as I shared with them first hand information from my personal experience and gave them support and encouragement. They were all extremely grateful. Three days later, he underwent surgery and has since made a full recovery.

HELPING OTHERS CAN GIVE ONE ENORMOUS SATISFACTION

Since that talk, I have been able to discuss and share my journey of fear and emotion with numerous other people suffering from similar problems as mine. Being able to share my experience made their road ahead become a lot clearer to understand and easier to cope with. I often wished that there had been such a person to talk to when I had to face that unknown journey.

Knowing just a little about that dark journey ahead of time can certainly help one to navigate that road a lot easier.

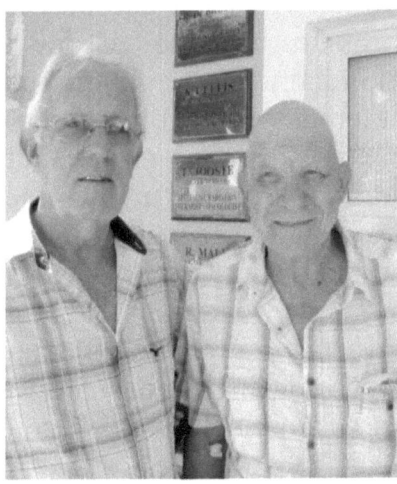

My mate Alan Dicks & I outside the clinic, we went through our treatments together.

My last chemo-radiation treatment finally ended on Tuesday 8th December 2009, after twenty five visits. It was a wonderful feeling to know that I would not have to make the daily trip to the hospital in the busy freeway traffic again. I had managed the treatments well and with minimum side effects during the entire twenty five sessions. Unfortunately many of the patients and new friends that I had made during the past few weeks did not have as easy a time as I had, with some of them suffering serious side effects. My mate Alan Dicks ended up in hospital with blood problems, luckily he was back in action a week later, this man is a fighter!

The psychological stress I felt seeing these people suffer on a daily basis during my five weeks of treatment was difficult for me to come to grips with and to fully understand.

The question that often comes up in my mind is the following. What if I had been for regular medical check-ups over the past few years with my General Practitioner, would my outcome have been any different? Would it have been possible to diagnose my problem much earlier? What if I had eaten less red meat during my lifetime and what if I had stayed out of the sun during my years as a farmer, would any of those changes have made my diagnosis any different? Would any of those changes have helped reduce the trauma that I had experienced during the past few weeks? Who knows, it's all history now.

HAVE A REGULAR MEDICAL CHECK UP

What I would like to suggest to readers from my experience is the following. I strongly recommend that you do yourself and your loved ones a big favour and have regular colon medical examinations. This is a quick and painless procedure which could save you a lot of unnecessary pain and suffering in the future if you took this precaution, it could save your life! In the event of a problem found, you will be diagnosed much earlier and could be in for a much easier time ahead.

Not many people have access to excellent free medical treatment these days therefore it is imperative that everyone should have an adequate Medical Insurance Plan, including hospitalization and cover for all major dreaded diseases. The cost of fighting cancer is astronomical!

In my opinion, I believe affordable medical care should be a right and not a luxury.

MEDICAL INSURANCE IS ESSENTIAL

Who knows what could be the cause of this dreaded disease called cancer, and when will medical science find a cure for it?

I have done a large amount of reading and research and my findings indicated that the following observations have been associated with the cause of cancer. These observations fall into two types of categories, namely <u>The Consumption of</u> and <u>The Exposure to.</u>

I have listed these results in total random order:

- High levels of stress

- Excessive protein and fat from meat and dairy products
- Excessive alcohol
- Excessive caffeine
- Excessive drugs
- Excessive cooked/processed foods
- Food preservatives
- Chemicals in drinking water
- Pesticides used in the food chain
- Tobacco products
- Toxic chemicals – air pollution, tobacco smoke, car exhaust fumes
- Radiation from Nuclear power stations, x-rays, exposure to the sun, high voltage overhead power lines

The question I keep asking myself is the following. Should you be lucky enough to survive major surgery, followed by all the chemotherapy and radiotherapy treatment, including all the dreadful side effects, what then does the Medical Profession have left to offer you as a cancer patient?

The answer I am sorry to say is nothing!

So, now where does one go from here and what does one do to try to keep healthy?

My finding showed that there are not too many options left for me to choose from. Once again, after a lot of research, I have found information that has given me some hope in this regard. Listed below is what I think looks to be the best options left for me to consider:

- Detoxification of your body after all the treatments
- Dietary changes in eating habits
- Supplement your body with additional vitamins and minerals
- Exercise for a healthy body

Many books are available covering these four subjects and therefore we would each need to structure our own individual plan. One would need to consult with an expert in each of these fields in order to arrive at what plan will suit you the best.

YOU WILL NEED TO CHANGE YOUR OLD HABITS

So what now is my plan you ask? Firstly, for me my diet is the most important item to start with. Dietary fats consumed from red meat and dairy products are by all accounts very bad news!

An interesting article I recently discovered showed that the human intestinal system is designed completely different from that of a carnivorous animal. Carnivores have a digestive system that is in place to process large quantities of meat, whereas our human system is not. I have cut down on red meat to once or twice a month. That has been my number one priority. Having been a farmer, I have always consumed large quantities of red meat as it was always a feature on our daily lunch menu. Eating more fresh fruit will now become a priority. Mixed nuts and dried fruit, both of which have never been popular with me will now appear on my shopping list. You cannot go wrong with large quantities of fresh vegetables including chicken and fish dishes.

Your new diet is therefore very important in rebuilding new healthy cells in your body.

Secondly, I will need to consult with a Nutritionist to discuss supplementing my run down body, including my depleted immune system. My liver and colon will need revitalising with the correct vitamins and minerals. I will need to get all of these internal organs up and running and in tip-top condition again.

Thirdly, over the years I have kept myself fit on a regular basis, but will now need to place more effort in this department by increased daily walking and swimming.

YOU MAY EXPERIENCE PANIC WHEN YOU PLAN FOR THE FUTURE, YOU WILL NEED TO KEEP A COOL HEAD

In addition to all of these new dietary plans, the biggest adjustment I needed to make in my life was now living with a colostomy bag. If you think that is difficult to deal with you are wrong. It's really quite simple, get your mind and attitude right and handle it. Living with a colostomy bag is so much better than being six feet under!

On a personal note, firstly very few people will ever know that you have a colostomy bag, unless you choose to tell them. Secondly, I have been asked this specific question a few times and the answer is as follows, once you fully recover from surgery with time and understanding and with a positive attitude, you can again enjoy a mutually satisfying sexual relationship with your partner.

SHARPEN YOUR AWARENESS AND BE THANKFUL OF THE FACT THAT A SLENDER THREAD BINDS US TO LIFE

Since my surgery, I have spent endless hours searching my memory for clues from my past that may help me in understanding why I had this overwhelming fear of hospitals and doctors. Both my parents had passed away some years back and were not here to throw any light on my youth years. I was on my own to try to figure this one out.

What has eventually filtered back to me after searching my memory and is now quite clear goes all the way back to my early childhood. I could have been three or four years old at the time and was with my mother visiting a dentist, probably for the first time. I must have been petrified as I recall screaming my head off. The dentist asked my mother to leave the room, as he knew how to calm me down. I cannot see his face at all, but I can picture him telling me to shut the hell up or he would stuff cotton wool down my throat! I have replayed this event over and over in my mind and

I am convinced that it was the start of my lifelong fear of doctors and hospitals.

KEEP THINKING POSITIVE THOUGHTS AND ONLY FOCUS FORWARD

The following morning, Wednesday 9th December 2009, Linda and I travelled six hundred kilometres to Johannesburg by car for a well earned two week holiday with our family. Once there we enjoyed the peace and tranquillity of their magnificent garden whilst lazing around their three swimming pools. For the first time in weeks I was able to erase from my mind the nightmare journey I had travelled during the past 100 days. Rest was the order of the day for me with plenty of time allocated to reading and sleeping.

One week after my last chemo-radiation treatment I could eventually take my first shower. I had clearly marked my diary for 16th December, my first shower in 42 days! The feeling was nothing short of awesome.

After a wonderful and restful 14 days in Johannesburg which had done me the world of good, we undertook the long return journey home, only three days before Christmas Day. We had to join the thousands of holiday makers on the busy freeway back to Durban, all making their way down to the many popular costal resorts for their annual holidays.

The best Christmas present that I have ever received in my life was on Christmas Eve, 24th

December 2009. I was sitting in the rooms of my Oncologist Dr Mall. He had just completed my physical examination and was about to give me the results of blood samples that had been taken the previous day.

"Mr Krebser, you are in great condition after your treatment. Your holiday has done you the world of good and you have even picked up a bit of weight. I am very pleased to tell you that the results of your full blood count (FBC) is perfectly normal, your liver function test (LFT) is normal and your tumour marker tests (CEA & CA199) are normal. I am very happy with these results, you are doing extremely well", he said.

Ecstatic was not the word. I was on cloud nine with excitement as I headed home at speed to share my good news with Linda, my family and close friends.

A date was later set for my follow up chemotherapy treatments to start from the first week in January 2010. I will continue on Xeloda tablets, as I had done well on them during my earlier chemo-radiation sessions.

The one unknown factor that I was now about to face, was the dosage of the drug was going to be stepped up from 1650mg per day taken during my radiotherapy treatments to 5300mg per day.

Was I going to cope with this increased dosage? I was going to have to swallow twelve tablets a day split into two daily sessions of six tablets each. The course would consist of an initial six sessions of three weeks each, or 18 weeks in total. Each session would consist of two weeks of chemo tablets followed by one week of rest and recovery. During these sessions my Oncologist would monitor my progress at the end of the third rest week with a physical examination and a detailed check on all my blood results.

I just hope my body holds up to the pounding the chemotherapy is about to give me. Should the oral form of treatment become far too difficult for me to handle, then we may elect to change my treatment to the drip format, which will require a trip to the clinic again once a week.

I am looking forward to the completion of this long journey of fear and emotion when I stand on top of the Highest Mountain Peak and scream aloud,

"Clear! - I am clear of cancer"

Remember, cancer is not an automatic death sentence! You will need to fight it. You will need to conquer the disease in the face of what appears to be those overwhelming odds against you.

YOU MUST NEVER EVER GIVE UP!

Finally, when you lie awake in those long dark hours of the night and your mind is racing in the wrong direction, as I often found mine doing, find strength in the following quotes:

"GET YOUR MIND RIGHT"

"TACKLE YOUR EMOTIONS"

"GET YOUR ATTITUDE RIGHT"

"FACE YOUR FEARS HEAD ON"

"NEVER, NEVER, NEVER GIVE UP"

Until then we wait, we watch, we monitor, we hope and we pray.

I am grateful each day that I am still alive!

Chapter Fourteen

Linda's Story

Ifirst met Eldred when I was a young girl in my teens. Our parents were friends so it was so natural for us also to become friends. From the time we met, I always knew that Eldred and I would be the best of friend because we had so much in common.

His schooling years were spent at a private boarding school in Johannesburg where he was a very astute student and an extremely good sportsman, particularly on the athletic field. For three years in succession, he won the "Victor Ludorum" trophy for outstanding athletic achievements. He achieved at everything he partook in and this was to be an accolade to follow him through his life.

After qualifying in Accountancy, he joined a well known Banking Group and eventually worked himself up through the ranks and became a bank teller. This is where Eldred discovered that he had a natural head for figures (both kinds).

Ambition led him to seek another job. He joined a very large Construction Company, listed on the Johannesburg Stock Exchange, running one of their subsidiary group companies. He worked himself up through the ranks from Accountant to

Company Secretary and eventually onto the Board of Directors. He later became the Chairman of the groups Inland Division responsible for all major civil engineering contracts. He spent 17 years with this company.

The "rat race" can become the most stressful thing for anyone to endure. We cannot all just pack our bags and move on, but Eldred had different ideas and decided he wanted to go farming and to spend the rest of his life in an entirely different environment. His family had farming roots in the country, going back as far as his grandfather's days in the early 1900's. Farming was in his blood!

Off he went to East Griqualand at the foothills of the Drakensburg Mountain Range to go cattle farming. Those years were not easy. Being under the African sun, wide open spaces and fresh air was the best thing anyone could ever wish for, especially after being in the city ones whole life. This farming stint lasted 20 years and he had relatively no stress at all. It was a good life style and he revelled in this hard but totally different way of life. He was the envy of many friends. Naturally he became a member of the Cricket, Tennis and Bowling Clubs and if he was not at some school sports day with one of the children, he was on one of the sports fields.

Eldred and I have spent the last five years in the wild African bush managing Game Farms. The life style has been amazing for us and we have enjoyed every minute of it. Eldred has always been fit and strong and never had to see a doctor for anything other than the normal eye tests and dental checkups.

We recently moved back to Durban due to unforeseen circumstances, and we constantly both crave to go back to the bush.

In the middle of last year 2009, for the first time ever, Eldred started to complain about his health, particularly pains in his stomach. This was most unusual and after about two days my first question to him was "Has your stomach worked" to which he replied, "No, I seem to be constipated". I went off to the local pharmacy and bought a laxative for him. Everything seemed to be alright. A few days later he complained of the same pains in his stomach and we went through the same procedure once again. He stopped complaining but to me he did not look well at all.

I remember mentioning this fact to the children and said I was worried about "Pops" which is the name all the children and grandchildren call him. I told them that this problem of his keeps recurring and that I suspected that he had a Bleeding Ulcer. They wished me good luck in trying to get him to see a doctor because even the suggestion of a doctor was just not negotiable to him and they knew how he felt about doctors.

We went through the same routine once again a few days later, this time with suppositories, Eldred was now in serious pain and discomfort and he complained his stomach felt like a ton of bricks. He had not had any bowel movement in days. This was most unusual for him. The medication worked to a certain degree but the pain was still there.

I was now starting to worry and suggested that he see a doctor as it was very clear to me that the problem was not going to go away with the medication we were using. At the mention of a doctor, he just clammed up and I could have been speaking to a brick wall with the amount of response I got.

He continued to complain for a few more days and I took no notice of him at all. However I was now becoming angry and eventually I told him in no uncertain terms that if he did not consult a doctor I did not want to hear another peep out of him. The complaining was to stop there and then.

This is something I can never understand about most men. If a woman has any sort of problem, we just take ourselves off to the doctor and sort the problem out with no fuss or worry. I am sure that any woman reading this book would agree with me on this matter. Men however cause all sorts of problems and complain until it is either too late or the problem becomes twice as large.

I believe that at this point, Eldred could see that I was very serious and fed up. This is when he decided to pay a visit to my GP Dr Yunus Motala, without telling me of course.

After receiving the news from Dr Motala that there was a possible restriction, he immediately drove to my work place to tell me the news. I was so relieved that he had seen the Doctor - I just had to say "I told you so".

Not for one moment did I ever think that it could be anything as serious as a cancerous tumour.

The following few days were somewhat ex-hausting as Eldred and I waited for the diagnosis, after he had gone through all the procedures required to know exactly what this restriction was!

We were sitting in the day clinic at the hospital waiting. Eldred was extremely nervous, his hands were clammy and he was very quiet while we waited for him to go into theatre to have the colonoscopy procedure. After what seemed like forever, the porter and theatre nurse arrived to take him to the theatre. He turned to me, squeezed my hand and said "Bye babe, please be here when I come back" in a very soft and shaky voice.

While he was in theatre, I was like a cat on a hot tin roof, pacing up and down the corridor, in and out of the ward just in case he came back. I tried to read a magazine but found myself continuously reading the same paragraph. I was not able to concentrate as my mind was in an absolute turmoil.

Eventually after what seemed like hours, the hospital staff wheeled him back into the ward. He was awake but I could see that he was non compus mentis. He kept telling me he was starving and needed something to eat. I ordered him sandwiches and tea as he slipped back into a deep sleep.

Dr Goga came into the ward to speak to me. He told me the procedure went well but "It does not look good at all," he said. He requested that we see him the following day in his consulting rooms to get the results of the tests he had sent to the laboratory. What did that mean? I was even more concerned and worried now. What was I going to say to Eldred when he woke up?

In a state of total confusion and shock, I just sat there with all sorts of things going through my mind and I was desperately trying to have positive thoughts. The sandwiches and tea arrived and he was so excited to see food that he took one bite out of each quarter, dropped one on the floor and then insisted on going home.

He was still a little confused as we made our way home. I never said anything to him about what Dr Goga had told me because I felt we first needed to see the test results. I did not want to cause any unnecessary anxiety. I never slept a wink that night.

The following day seemed to drag as our appointment with Dr Goga was only at 2pm. When we arrived at his rooms, we were immediately ushered into his office. We sat down and after the initial greeting's, Dr Goga looked at Eldred and said, "Mr Krebser, I am very sorry to tell you this. I have discovered a tumour approximately 5cm in length in your colon and from the biopsy I had taken and the test results, it is cancerous. I'm so sorry to have to tell you this bad news".

Dr Goga continued to speak as I looked at Eldred and saw the colour drain from his face. I felt numb as I tried to grasp what we had just been told. I could not even imagine what Eldred was feeling. I am sure that no one knows exactly how a person feels after learning that one has cancer unless you have been there. At that very moment I could feel his pain and fear as he took my hand and looking into my eyes and deep down into my soul, he was asking for help without saying a word. We both had tears rolling down our cheeks. I realised at that moment that I now had to be stronger than I had ever been before.

We left the doctor's rooms and spent the next hour looking for our car. It was exactly where we had left it. It is amazing what shock can do to one's mind in the heat of the moment. Once we found the car the first person I phoned was Dawn our daughter who had phoned while we were in with the doctor. I had promised to return the call as soon as we left his rooms. When I heard her voice I was unable to speak and passed the phone to Eldred. He conveyed the bad news and she was devastated. She is very close to her Pops. I then phoned Amy, our very dear friend who was diagnosed with breast cancer a few months earlier. All I could say to her was "Amy, we have just been given the results, and it is not good. Please we need your help"

We had only been home a short while when she arrived. Amy was a tower of strength for both of us as she is a very calm and rational person. She explained all sorts of procedures that could happen in the months to come. It was the fear of the unknown that we could not come to terms with. She shed light on many unanswered questions which somehow made everything a lot easier to cope with.

By this time I had calmed down enough to phone all the children with the news of their father.

They all took it quite badly. Understandably it was a huge shock to everyone. I had to keep reminding myself that I had to be their pillar of strength.

We now had to prepare ourselves for the surgery which was Eldred's biggest fear.

I clearly remember the day we checked into the hospital. At first he was very quiet, but as the minutes ticked by he became very talkative and I think that the other three men in the ward must have thought that this man had done the hospital thing many times before. On the outside he seemed so confident. He told them all it was a walk in the park and they should not worry about a thing and that everything would be just fine. I was amazed, but I knew it was merely a front and that deep down he was petrified.

Once all the paper work was completed and he had seen all the nurses, doctors and therapists it was time for him to proceed to the theatre for this very serious operation. In a heartbeat Eldred once again became very quiet. I assured him that all would be fine, as I would stay with him till he entered the theatre. He held my hand so tightly that it stopped the circulation and all I could feel was numbness! I stayed with him until they took him into theatre.

Suddenly I felt very alone. My man was going under the knife to have this terrible disease removed from his body. "Please dear God look after my man", I prayed. I sat in the hospital for more than five hours waiting. After what seemed like a lifetime, they wheeled him through the doors where I had been waiting patiently. He had pipes coming out of every part of his body and I could see that even though he seemed awake, he was not with me.

In the Intensive Care Unit, they made him comfortable before they would let me in. When I entered the unit he was bright eyed and greeted me with a smile as if nothing had happened. This was short lived as he drifted off into a deep sleep. The sister sent me home to return the following day as he was on Morphine and not coherent. I returned home to spend my birthday alone as none of our children live anywhere close.

I remembered that I had not eaten the whole day and was famished. While pondering on what I should have for dinner, the gate bell rang and there was my very special friend Colleen who had come to spend the night and to share my birthday with me. We had special quality time together that evening chatting about all sorts. This kept my mind off just how depressed and down I was.

I slept well that night for the first time in weeks. Colleen was my lifesaver that evening even though she did not know it at the time.

The following morning I was at the hospital bright and early but was only allowed into the ICU at 11am. I was most surprised to find Eldred looking so much better. He had colour back in his face and seemed quite chirpy. I was not sure what to expect from him but was amazed at his attitude. He was positive and so badly wanted to get well and get out of hospital as quickly as possible. It was then that I realized that he was going to come through all this with flying colours. We just needed to work on his recovery. I was determined to keep him in good spirits.

After two and a half days in ICU he was transferred to a general ward where he went from strength to strength. However he did have to overcome a few emotional moments. I was now convinced that he was over the worst.

The day I brought him home was Sunday 27th September 2009. That was the day he told me he was going to write a book about his fears, emotions and his journey through this terrifying time in his life. I thought it was a brilliant idea and gave him my full support and encouragement.

It was good to have him home!

After going through the chemo-radiation and then the harsh dosages of chemo therapy, we have come a long way. Eldred has coped exceptionally well through these really hard and trying times. For me it has not been easy because he has had terrible mood swings and at times been really nasty. I have tried very hard and believe that the worst is almost over. The person closest always bears the brunt and needs to be strong at all times. There have been moments when I have wanted to run away and never come back, but I am a very strong and level headed person so I have persevered and coped. I will not allow anything to get the better of me and will stay in control of my emotions. After all, this is my man, my soul mate and the person I will grow old with. I am so proud of him and I love him dearly.

At times, the last six months seems to have been a bad dream but then reality strikes and there is no dream at all.

We have since spent many hours together making plans for our immediate future. We are a great team together and at our daily "Board Meeting", plans are in place to spend quality time doing things that we have often only dreamt about.

Life is so unpredictable. We are going to make our dreams come true while we are still able to. Writing this book has been so good for Eldred. It has kept his mind busy over the past months and created some meaning in his life. I hope you enjoy reading this book and I am glad that it is now complete.

Linda, Durban, Feb 2010

Postscript
In Diary Format

Chemo - Half Way (12/3/2010)

The date today is 12th March 2010 and it's my 62nd birthday. My surgery took place on Linda's birthday 21/9/09 and my book ended 6 months later on my birthday, quite uncanny.

I am half way there! This week I have managed to complete the ninth week of my eighteen weeks of chemotherapy treatment. Other than very sore feet (foot syndrome) and slight nausea, both side effect of the chemo, I am doing really well.

Great news today! I have had my half way check up including Blood tests, Ultrasound of my abdomen and a chest X-Ray and the results have all been positive. I have passed with flying colours! It's difficult to explain what I am feeling now – such a great relief after all the hardship. Nine weeks to go......

Chemo -Complete (12/5/2010)

We have now reached the completion of my 18 weeks of Chemotherapy and I can report to the readers that I have again passed all the required tests with flying colours. My bloods, ultrasound and x-rays have all come back with positive excellent results. Other than occasional bouts of mild nausea and hand foot syndrome I have somehow managed to get through the 18 weeks of Chemo extremely well. All those earlier fears of facing the terrible side effects of Chemotherapy are now over and hopefully something of the past. Again, one has no idea of my complete feeling of relief!

Support Group

During the past weeks I was invited to join a new Cancer Support Group which was being formed in our neighbourhood. The first meeting attracted 50 local people, most of whom were cancer sufferers and their supporters. What a privilege it was when asked to address the second meeting and share with all present my personal journey of fear, emotion and the subsequent writing of my book "Cancer, Thirty One Days"

Through my Doctor, Surgeon and press releases in the local media I have had the privilege of speaking to and assisting numerous cancer patients both pre and post operative. To have been able to speak to and assist just one person in facing his or her fears has been a great leveller for me.

Cancer Association of South Africa

In July 2010 my book was officially recognised and approved by the Cancer Association of South

Africa. It has now been made available to the general public and can be viewed on their official website www.cansa.org.za

For every book sold, I will donate a portion of the proceeds from the sale to Cansa, to help in promoting their cause. I am grateful to them for their recognition and support.

Netcare Hospital Group

I am also grateful to the Netcare Hospital Group in South Africa for embracing the content and spirit of my book and making it available to Cancer patient's country wide through their vast network of Hospitals and Oncology Units. I thank them for their help and involvement

Finally (Sept 2010)

It is time for the book, "Cancer, Thirty One Days" to come to an end.

I however will not come to an end - I will never ever give up fighting.

Finally in conclusion, I live each day with thankfulness and I thank God each day that I am still alive!

"Never, never, never, give up"

Sir Winston Churchill

"All battles are first won or lost in the mind"

Joan of Arc

SPECIAL THANKS

I would like to express my sincere gratitude and thanks to the following people, without whom I may not have been here to tell my story:-

Dr Yunus Motala – General Practitioner. Yunus, thank you for swiftly referring me to a Specialist Surgeon. Your concern for my health will always be appreciated.

Dr Anver Goga – Specialist Surgeon. Anver, thank you for saving my life! Also to your colleagues, the Surgeons and Medical Team who assisted you.

Dr M A Laher & Dr Ruwaida Khan - Specialist Anaesthesiologists. You took me on a long dark journey and brought me back alive.

Dr Riaz Mall – Specialist Oncologist.Riaz, thank you for giving me inspiration, courage, support and hope to prolong my life. Thanks also to Dr Rob de Bruyne and your efficient staff at Hopelands Cancer Centre.

Life Westville Hospital – The Intensive Care Unit and Ward Sisters for their efficient & dedicated nursing care.

Netcare Parklands Hospital – The Radiotherapy staff. Ashni, Tina and Merridy, thanks for those 25 efficient treatments.

Sister Jocelyn Taylor – My Stomatherapist. Thanks Jocelyn for your advice & support. Life with a Colostomy is now so much easier to live with.

Pete Kruger & Jerome Moses – Thanks to you both for continually picking me up when I was down. I value your friendship.

To my Family and Friends – The list will take up another book, but you all know who you are. To every one of you, a very big Thank You.

The following people are **very important in my life** and I need to make special mention of them:

Gregory & Dawn - Wayne & Lisa - Bruce & Charnelle - Chris & Kim - Paul & Debbilee - all 13 of my grandchildren – Tyler – Bailey - Dennis – Connor – Kyle – Georgia – Keira – Rhylie – Robin – Dakota – Lex – Kayla – Ella - my brother Noel – Sandy – Sherilyn – Heather – my cousin Sonia - very special friends Angela - Pete & Wendy - Ahmed & Amy - Colleen and my friendly neighbours Brian, Dorothy and Chris.

Thanks to all of you for your love, encouragement, hospital visits, home visits, phone calls, emails, prayers and never ending support, I thank you all from the bottom of my heart.

Finally, to the most important person in my life

Linda – My Partner and best friend, you are the light in my life that constantly shows me the way. Without your loving support and encouragement, I could never ever have coped throughout this, the most traumatic and terrifying time in my life. I deeply value your love.

With all my love,

EK.

SEQUENCE OF EVENTS

Wednesday, 26 August 2009
>   Dr Motala – Initial Diagnosis

Thursday, 27 August 2009
>   Dr Goga – Discussed procedure

Tuesday, 1 September 2009
>   Gastroscopy/Colonoscopy

Wednesday, 2 September 2009
>   Dr Goga – Cancer Diagnosis

Tuesday, 8 September 2009
>   Dr Mall – Oncologist

Wednesday, 9 September 2009
>   Ultrasound

Thursday, 10 September 2009
>   Dr Mall – Results

Wednesday, 16 September 2009
>   MRI Scan

Thursday, 17 September 2009
>   Dr Goga – Surgery discussion

Monday, 21 September 2009
>   Linda's Birthday – Surgery

Tuesday & Wednesday, 22/23 September 2009

  Intensive Care Unit

Thursday, 24 September 2009

  Intensive Care Unit/Ward

Friday & Saturday, 25/26 September 2009

  Ward

Sunday, 27 September 2009

  Ward/Home

Monday, 5 October 2009

  Staples out

Monday, 12 October 2009

  Dr Goga – Post op physical

Wednesday, 14 October 2009

  Dr Mall – The Road ahead

Wednesday, 21 October 2009

  Radiotherapy set-up

Wednesday, 4 November 2009

  Chemo-radiation No 1

Tuesday, 8 December 2009

  Chemo-radiation No 25

Email address

thirtyonedays@webmail.co.za

Website address

www.cancer-thirtyonedays.com

A portion of the sale

of this book

will be donated to The

Cancer Association of South Africa.